AF359481

TABLE OF CONTENTS

Dedication

Gratitude & Acknowledgements

Introduction

Hey there! Hope you are doing great! I thank you for buying this book unless you are still checking it out and wondering if this book is for you! If so, then let me clear your doubts. This won't be a typical weight loss book, dear. There are no diet charts. As I do not wake up early morning, I choose not to write about effective morning routines and schedules. No food and drinks that make you Lose Weight Fast. No heavy workouts. No cardio. No screaming gym trainers. No family members pushing you to lose weight.

So, what is this book about? What's in it for me?
This book is about creating those tiny and magnificent shifts in your heart, in your mind and in your being to help you create more ease towards achieving your weight loss goal. The techniques in this book aim to create more lightness and joy by reducing the emotional stress and pressure to lose weight.

How Does it Work?
As you learn to apply the Emotional Freedom Technique towards your specific weight loss challenge, chapter by chapter, you start peeling off those unhealthy thoughts and emotions that keep you away from losing weight. These unhealthy thoughts and emotions are present beneath the physical weight in the form of demands you put on yourself, guilt, emotional overwhelm, frustration, impatience, poor self-image, judgements and fears. It is this emotional weight and the unaddressed issues that lead to binge eating, stress eating, reduced control over your diet, procrastination tendencies and inconsistent actions thereby

causing you to gain weight rather than lose it. This book provides EFT solutions, towards these specific issues, thereby reducing the intensity of these issues. Consider this book as a friend who is talking to you every day and taking off the weight of losing weight from your shoulders. Resolving one problem every day. Making progress slowly but surely.

What Is EFT & What to Expect?

EFT stands for Emotional Freedom Technique, also known as tapping. It is a mind-body technique meant to clear emotional blocks. This technique involves tapping with your fingertips. It is a form of psychological acupressure based on the ancient principle of acupuncture, except that it does not use needles. While focusing on the issue, you are supposed to tap on the specific body points and speak out loud about your issue like you are talking to your friend. It's so easy! To make it easier, I have included suggestions on what you can say about specific issues.

Each time you complete the tapping, you can measure the intensity of your issue before and after and notice the positive change in your emotional well-being. Expect a shift in your consciousness with self-love and self-acceptance. Be more comfortable with your present body and weight and pursue your weight-loss goal with more ease, joy, and enthusiasm. Truly expect to Lighten Up!

My Weight Loss Story!

Just like you, I too have tried innumerable diet plans, consulted several dieticians and wasted a lot of money going to the gym. Created weight loss goals & did not achieve them. Had many weight loss resolutions that failed miserably. I did manage to lose about 35 pounds at a point in my life and then gained 30 as well. My weight loss journey has been equally difficult. Presently I do not consider myself to be perfectly fit however I am much more at ease about my body, my image and myself. I still do not like when my old clothes don't fit in. I still feel uncomfortable during social gatherings and I too dream of having a great body. While I continue to dream about this, I discovered that I can be a lot easy on myself for achieving this goal. Being easy on yourself does not mean being lazy or any less committed. I take care of myself well. I eat fruits, I do my dancing for about 30-40 minutes on awesome dance tracks, I eat consciously, do EFT tapping for my weight. After a long day at work, if I don't have the stamina to dance, I go for a walk. Sometimes I do not have the energy even to walk, I sit back home and watch Netflix over a cup of coffee and enjoy the relaxation time. I don't feel guilty about missing out on my dance or walks as I acknowledge that some days are mentally very difficult and my mind and body need that additional pampering during those days. At work, when my office friends order food (junk food) from outside I do join them but I do not overeat. I intend to lose 35 pounds but I won't starve or punish myself mentally, emotionally or physically. I am progressing towards achieving my weight goal by simply being more aware and mindful of the actions that I need to do to lose weight. I have realized that planning my day i.e., TODAY and intending to do the activities that help me lose weight is a far easier and more practical approach than setting monthly goals and not achieving them. I look at myself in the mirror and I feel more comfortable than before. Am I entirely happy with my body and weight? NO. Am I doing what it takes to lose weight?

YES. Am I easy on myself to achieve my goal, definitely YES. Do I still experience unhealthy emotions like anger, cravings, regret and frustration about losing weight? YES, I do. But now I quickly lower the intensity of these emotions with tapping. I focus on what I am supposed to do. I do not stay for a long time in these unhealthy thoughts and emotions. This choice to no longer stay in these emotions comes with awareness and practising EFT. So, if you too want to get rid of those unhealthy and draining emotions that are holding you back from losing weight, then I welcome you with a warm and compassionate heart to the world of EFT. Re-start your weight-loss journey with more lightness, calmness and confidence. A renewed self, oozing in self-love, self-care and acceptance.

Am grateful to have learnt EFT and also grateful to my clients, while working on their weight loss issues, my issues also got resolved. Here are some of the inspiring feedbacks my clients gave after they experienced the positive changes from EFT.

Client's Speaking From their Heart!

My belief about building a positive image has shifted greatly. I have started to accept myself now. My body had become rigid in these years; however, after the EFT sessions, I have restarted my yoga practice, and my body is much more flexible now.

I just attended a session on weight loss with Kunal Dudeja. It helped me let go of my fears that I am old to lose weight and accept my body. The workshop helped with the release of hidden subconscious emotions. I look forward to being motivated to achieve my exercise goals daily. Thank you so much, Kunal!

It's been 4 days since I did EFT on the tapping script on stress and anxiety. For the last 4 days, I did not get any cravings or urge to jump to sweets. My mind is relaxed too. I thank you, Kunal for this beautiful script. In measurable terms, my craving for food reduced from a 9 to a 3 on a scale of 10.

In today's session, I felt a significant shift in me. I could relate my sugar craving to the stress levels from the last 6 months, resulting from work pressure, relationship issues and financial instability. Felt like something got released from my body. My stress intensity has reduced from 9/10 to 4/10. My sleep pattern has improved. Sugar cravings reduced from 9/10 to 5/10.

I attended online zoom sessions for weight loss with Kunal and I can't explain with what ease he conducts them and the shifts. I could feel the shifts in my emotions be it anxiety, fear or disbelief. The best part was that it motivated me to start my walks and I did begin immediately. I now believe that I can lose weight, and if this belief shakes up then I have EFT to my rescue.

Hello Kunal, today, I am short of words to express my gratitude to you. Today's EFT for working on a belief system, connecting to the events and the EFT forgiveness was superb. I could easily connect to where I picked the beliefs and how I tried to fit in with other people's perceptions and visions. I not only tried to fit in but also made it my own. It was a great insight into how I lived all these years to other people's beliefs and how I continued to carry and live with family beliefs. With your prompt EFT guidance, it was so unexpected that within a few rounds, my SUDS score went from a 10 on 10 to a 3 on 10.

Thank you, Kunal for the fantastic EFT workshop you have set up and for motivating me to take the first step towards a fitter mindset. This experience has left me feeling more empowered and confident that I can still lose the weight that I had put on post-pregnancy. Thank you for showing me my real power of mental strength. Through this experience, I have learnt so much more about myself and how repeating the same things makes me look petty. Thank you so much for being so good at what you do. Even when we were in the group, you were observing each one of us which is commendable. You have such a beautiful practice, and I admire your confidence in all you do and say, of course with a smile. And last but not least, I thank you for teaching me to live life and love myself the way I am and tap the anxiety and phobia of weight loss out of my life.

My experience of having food after the session was excellent. I have had the habit of just swallowing the food since my childhood. By the time the other members of my family start eating, my dinner is almost over. But tonight, when I sat for dinner, I took a full 15 minutes to complete it. For the first time, I could feel the taste of my food. My teeth chew food after ages. Most important is the quantity of food I ate was half of my everyday meal. What a shift!

Disclaimer

This book does not provide any medical advice nor prescribe any technique to treat physical, emotional, mental, and medical problems. For any such issues, you are required to consult your physician, counsellor or mental health practitioner as you consider appropriate. This book intends to offer information of a generic nature for your spiritual evolution. If you use any of the book's information for yourself, the author and the publisher assume no responsibility for your actions. The reader of this book must take complete responsibility for its use. Further, the author offers the information in this book solely as his opinion. Readers are strongly cautioned and advised to consult a licensed healthcare professional before using any of the information in this book. The author, publisher and contributors of this book and other parties related (a) explicitly disclaim any liability for and shall not be liable for any loss or damage including but not limited to use of this information; (b) shall not be liable for any direct or indirect compensatory, special, incidental, or consequential damages or costs of any kind or character; (c) shall not be responsible for any acts or omission by any party including but not limited to any party mentioned or included in the information or otherwise (d) do not endorse or support any material or information from any party mentioned or included in the information or otherwise(e) will not be liable for damages or costs resulting from any claim whatsoever. If the reader or user does not agree with any of the foregoing terms, the reader or user should not use the information in this book to read it. A reader who continues reading this book will be deemed to have accepted the provisions of this disclaimer.

Part 1

Lighten Up Your Knowledge

Chapter 1

Learning Emotional Freedom Technique

Hey there! Excited to learn EFT? I am sure you are, so let us dive into it. The Emotional Freedom Technique is been well-known to create effective results since its introduction by Gary Craig in the 1990s. It is a gentle touch with your fingertips on specific body points, coupled with the power of your intention, that can create miraculous results. By the end of this chapter, you will learn the basics of EFT and create an open mind to apply EFT for your weight loss issues.

What is EFT or Tapping?

EFT stands for Emotional Freedom Technique, also known as tapping. It is a mind-body technique meant to clear emotional blocks. This technique involves tapping with your fingertips. It is a form of psychological acupressure based on the ancient principle of acupuncture, except that it does not use needles. EFT combines gentle tapping with your fingertips on key acupuncture points while focusing on the issue. Once you have completed tapping on the various points, the intensity of the emotional charge of the issue reduces. EFT is easy to understand and apply and very easy to measure the results.

Location of EFT Tapping Points

Karate Chop Point (KC): This point is in the middle of the fleshy part of the hand's outside edge. You can tap with four fingers of the opposite hand on this point.

Beginning of Eyebrow (EB): Located at the beginning of the eyebrow, just above and to one side of the nose.

Side of Eye (SE): Located on the outside of the eye socket near the outside corner of the eye.

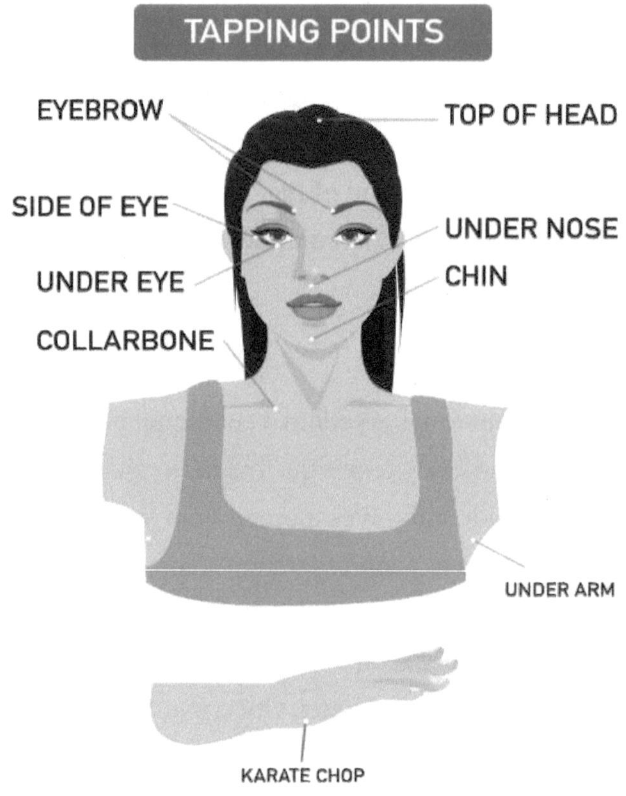

Under the Eye (UE): Located on the bone underneath the eye, approximately 1 inch below the pupil.

Under Nose (UN): Located between the nose and the upper lip.

Chin (CH): Located between the lower lip and chin.

Collarbone (CB): This point is located on the inner edge of the collarbone. Just an inch or two from the center towards the left or right. This point is where you will feel a slight indentation on your collarbone.

Under Arm (UA): Located at the side of the body. About four inches down from the armpit.

Tapping with all the Fingers & Thumb (AFT)
Tap using both the hand's fingertips and thumb with each other.

Top of Head (ToH): Located directly in the centre on top of the head. When tapping on the top of your head, use all your fingertips.

The Set-Up Statement
A set-up statement is a self-acceptance statement combined with the description of the issue. It begins with the words "Even Though", and then the person is supposed to describe the problem and follow it up with a love and acceptance statement or a choice statement like "I accept myself" or "I deeply and completely love and accept myself" or I choose to heal now. The format of the setup is **Even Though, <Describe the issue>, I <State the Love & Acceptance statement or the Choice statement>.**

Examples of set-up statements

- Even though I have no enthusiasm for losing weight, I accept myself.
- Even though I eat food to heal my sadness, I love and accept myself.
- Even though I have no control over food, I accept and love myself.
- Even though I feel ashamed when I look at myself in the mirror, I deeply and completely accept myself.
- Even though food comforts me when I am anxious, I accept myself and choose to relax now.
- Even though I fear that I will gain back the weight I have lost; I choose to love and accept myself.
- Even though I have this intense craving to eat these chips, I allow myself to relax
- Even though I feel lazy to go the gym, I choose to hit the gym anyway
- Even though I find it difficult to let go of this guilt, I choose to release this emotion with love
- Even though my past failure has shaken my level of confidence, I love myself and choose to regain my confidence
- Even though I binge eat these chips and I cannot control it, I accept how I feel and choose to create healthy eating habits
- Even though I am frustrated with my weight & body, I choose to love and accept myself
- Even though I have no patience to lose weight, I choose to relax and create joyful patience.
- Even though I do not know if I can lose any pounds, I accept myself and choose to think of possibilities of losing weight.

Awesome examples correct?

You are supposed to say the entire set-up statement while you tap on the Karate Chop point at least 3-4 times for the specific issues you are working on.

Reminder Phrases

These are those words or phrases that are related to the problem you intend to resolve. Examples of reminder phrases in connection with weight loss could be "It is so difficult to lose weight", "I have tried several times, and I have failed", "I cannot control my sweet craving", "I do not know how to lose weight" and so on.

Reminder phrases are to be said while tapping on all the points – Eyebrow (EB), Side of Eye (SE), Under Eye (UE), Under Nose (UN), Chin (CH), Collarbone (CB), Under Arm (UA), All Fingers & Thumb (AFT), and Top of Head (ToH).

Tapping Count and Fingers

Tap 7-8 times on each tapping point using your index, middle and ring finger. You can use a broader coverage for the top of the head, collarbone, and underarms. When you tap, you may be inclined to stay longer on some points, whereas on some, a shorter time. Go by your intuition.

Tapping Ways

You can tap on either side of the body. For example, you could do one round on one side of the body and the other on the other. You could use your left hand to tap or your right hand. You can also use both hands when you tap too.

Tapping Pressure

Tap firmly, but not so hard that you may hurt yourself or leave some bruises. Certainly, go easy on the side of the eye and top of the head as those are more delicate parts of the tapping points.

EFT Tapping Methods

There are two methods of tapping:

Method 1 – Talk, Feel and Tap (Highly Recommended)

While you are tapping on the points, talk out loud about the issue you are working on. Talk as if you are expressing your problem to your friend. When you do this, you will be surprised how hidden emotions come up for tapping. This method is known as the "Tell the Story Method". It is like talking about your issue in the form of a story.

Method 2 – Think, Feel and Tap

As the name suggests, keep tapping while thinking about your problem. Think about the event or the person that has caused this issue. See what you see, hear what you hear and feel the emotions. Play the issue like a movie in your mind and keep tapping on the points. You can use this method when you do not wish to talk about your issue. If your issue's intensity is exceptionally high, you may want to speak to your therapist.

Tapping Sequence or Tapping Rounds

The tapping sequence starts with KC and is completed by tapping on the ToH. When tapping on the KC, you are to speak out loud the set-up statement 3-4 times. You can bring in variations when you speak your set-up statements. For all the other points, tap and talk about the specific issue you are working on. The tapping sequence is as below:

Karate Chop (KC) for Set Up Statements

Eyebrow (EB)

Side of Eye (SE)

Under Eye (UE)

Under Nose (UN)

Chin (CH)

Collarbone (CB)

Under Arm (UA)

All Fingers & Thumb (AFT)

Top of Head (ToH)

Tapping Script

Tapping scripts are guidelines, and you are free to modify the script based on your intuition. These are suggestions; on what words and phrases you can say while working on the issue. The scripts typically consist of 6-7 rounds. Depending on the intensity of your issue, you could tap less or more. The format of the scripts is kept very simple.

For initial rounds, you tap on the setup statement (KC) and reminder phrases. Once your SUDS score reduces, then you can tap on closing rounds which involves

- Tapping on all the points stating your problem statement
- Tapping on all the points stating your love and acceptance or choice statement
- Tapping on all the points alternating between your problem statement and love and acceptance statement.

In these closing rounds, choose the most appropriate problem and love and acceptance statement to tap on. Don't worry! I have included plenty of tapping scripts for several issues. You will get a hang of it.

SUDS

SUDS stands for Subjective Unit of Distress Scale. It is a scale used to measure the subjective intensity of distress experienced by an individual about the issue. A score of 0 represents that there is no intensity or no distress. A score of 10 means that the issue's intensity is the highest. For high scores, kindly consult your therapist.

What to Speak During Tapping

You can talk about various aspects of the issue that you are working on. Do not limit talking about symptoms or the consequences of the issue. Talk about the underlying emotions, the past events or triggers and the belief systems you created about the issue. For example, you are having a headache. Maybe you are resisting speaking with your spouse and withholding your anger. Hence talk and tap about this resistance. Perhaps an event happened in the past that is creating this resistance. Hence talk about this event. Also, talk about the present belief you created because of this event. For example, *I should not speak what I feel, to protect myself.* Talk about this belief. You may notice, the deeper you dive into the issue, the faster you heal.

Close the Session

Once you have completed all the tapping rounds, sit by and relax, sip some water. Express gratitude to EFT and the founders. Make a note of your learnings, realizations or actions.

What to Expect Post Tapping

You may feel drowsy, thirsty, sleepy, fresh, tired, crying, sad, energetic, yawning, burping, or wanting to use the washroom. These are all signs of release and the shifts happening post the tapping. Side effects of tapping are that you could feel a sense of ease, a sense of freedom. You could feel happy and delighted too. You could lighten up.

Guidelines for Effective Tapping

1. Do not generalize your issue. Be specific about your issue.
2. When you tap, turn off or put your phone or put it on silent.
3. Wear comfortable clothes and find a relaxing place.
4. Remove any item that may hinder tapping, such as your eyeglasses, rings, or bracelets.
5. Drink water in between the tapping rounds.
6. Bring in some variations in the set-up statement. Be louder when you say it. Add or remove some words. Check on how you are feeling about the revised set-up statement.
7. Tune into the issue before tapping. It is important that you tune into the issue, before tapping for better results. Think about those events, situations, and emotions and go into your heart space to tune in. To tune in, you can say to yourself –

- I go into my heart space to feel this issue to heal it
- I now choose to bring up this issue for resolution
- I tune into this issue within my heart and so on

Summary of the Tapping Process

The tapping process is summarised as per the steps below:

1. Identify the specific issue which you intend to resolve and measure the SUDS score

2. Tap on the Karate chop point, repeating the set-up statements out loud 3 to 4 times.

3. Repeat the reminder phrases relating to your issue while you tap on the remaining points

4. Re-assess the intensity of your issue between the tapping rounds.

5. Keep talking about various aspects of your issue. The symptoms, underlying emotions, the events associated with it, and the belief systems. Express gratitude and close.

I highly recommend that you do not rush to finish reading this book. Apply the EFT or tapping solution to your weight loss issue, one at a time. Once the issue intensity has come down to an acceptable level, then move to the next chapter. It's best to work on one issue at one time (For example working on chocolate cravings) till the SUDS score comes down to a 2 or less and then move to other issues. Some issues could take a few days and several rounds of tapping. Be patient, and work on that issue only. Once it is resolved, you might just experience a breakthrough and other issues can be worked on easily.

Going The Extra Mile

While most of my clients are very happy when their SUDS score comes down to a 2 or a 1, some aren't. They want to get their SUDS score to zero. If you too feel that way, and despite tapping several rounds, if your SUDS is not getting to zero and is stuck at 1 or a 2, then you can do the 9 Gamut procedure. This 9-gamut procedure involves tapping on a point located on the back of the hand while focusing on the issue and going through 9 steps which involve eye movements, humming and counting.

First, locate the point on the back of the hand. It is about an inch down from the knuckles between the little finger and the ring finger. Next, find that space with one or more fingers of the opposite hand, moving from the knuckles toward the wrist until you feel a slight indentation. It feels like the right spot when you gently rub, hold, or tap there. Refer to the hand image to see the location of this point.

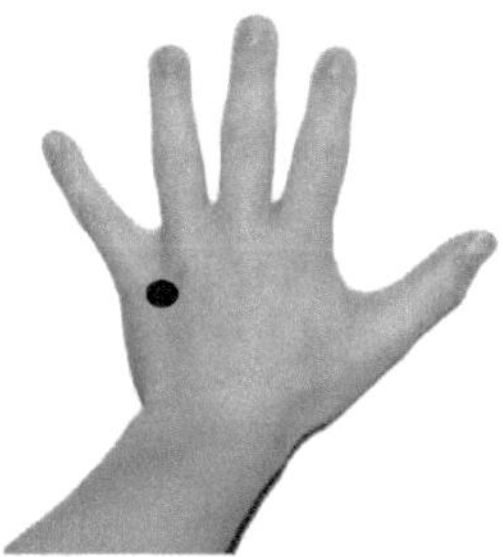

You are supposed to tap continuously on this point using two or more fingers of the opposite hand. However, I recommend using four fingers for excellent results. The 9-gamut procedure involves tapping on the gamut point while completing nine steps as listed below while you focus on the issue.

For each of the nine steps, keep tapping continuously on the gamut spot for approximately 4 to 5 seconds with your head still.

Step 1) Close your eyes.

Step 2) Open your eyes.

Step 3) Keeping your head still, look hard down to your right.

Step 4) Keeping your head still, look hard down to your left.

Step 5) Keeping your head still, roll your eyes in a full circle in one direction.

Step 6) Keeping your head still, roll your eyes in a full circle in the opposite direction.

Step 7) Hum any song out loud for 4 to 5 seconds. You can hum the happy birthday song.

Step 8) Quickly count aloud from 1 to 5 and then from 5 to 1.

Step 9) Hum the song for 4 to 5 seconds.

Even if you interchange the order of the steps when you are doing the gamut tapping, it is fine if you do all the steps. After completing steps 3, 4, 5 and 6, you can allow your eyes to come back into the central/normal position while tapping. I have noticed effective results for my clients when they do this.

So Far So Good?

I Love & Accept Myself

Chapter 2

Cultivating an Open Mind to Apply EFT

Now that you are familiar with how EFT works, let us practice it. If you are new to EFT or therapy work, you might have doubts and apprehensions. Questions like - *Whether this will work? Is this for real? Is it right for me?* may pop up. That's okay. We will implement EFT to calm the doubts and apprehensions about EFT itself. Sounds good? So, let us start.

Take three deep breaths and tune into these doubts and apprehensions about EFT. Make a mental note of the SUDS score *(Your SUDS score will be 0/10 if you are fully open to learning EFT. It will be a 10/10 if you are full of doubts & apprehensions)* about your openness to learn and use EFT, and start tapping and speaking out loud as below.

Round 1
KC: Even though I know nothing about EFT, I don't mind trying it.
KC: Even though I am unsure how EFT would help with my weight loss, I am open to exploring this possibility.
KC: Even though I believe I can lose weight only by diet and workouts, I am willing to learn something new.
EB: I have no clue whether this thing will work.
SE: I have my doubts and apprehensions about EFT
UE: Losing weight is difficult.
UN: Not sure how EFT would help me lose weight.

CH: This idea itself seems so weird.

CB: Will this work?

UA: This may be a waste of time.

AFT: <Talk about how you feel>

ToH: This is vague and uncertain

Round 2

EB: I am still not feeling much of a change.

SE: Am not sure if it is working.

UE: I doubt how the results will show up.

UN: Would tapping on my body create any change?

CH: I doubt if this technique can transform me.

CB: I have tried so many things in the past.

UA: Never heard or tried something like this before

AFT: <Talk about how you feel>

ToH: I will believe only if it gives me good results.

Take a pause and 3 deep breaths. Assess the SUDS score and make a note of it. Starting tapping as below:

Round 3

KC: Even though am not entirely convinced about EFT, there is no harm in trying it.

KC: Even though I still have some doubts, I accept myself and choose to be open to trying EFT.

KC: Even though it is not easy to lose weight just by tapping, am open towards the possibility of learning EFT

EB: <Talk about your doubts & apprehensions>

SE: <Talk about your doubts & apprehensions>

UE: <Talk about your doubts & apprehensions>

UN: <Talk about your doubts & apprehensions>
CH: <Talk about your doubts & apprehensions>
CB: <Talk about your doubts & apprehensions>
UA: <Talk about your doubts & apprehensions>
AFT: <Talk about your doubts & apprehensions>
ToH: <Talk about your doubts & apprehensions>

Round 4

Take a pause and a couple of breaths and start tapping.

EB: Even though I do not entirely believe in EFT.
SE: Even though I do not entirely believe in EFT.
UE: Even though I do not entirely believe in EFT.
UN: Even though I do not entirely believe in EFT.
CH: Even though I do not entirely believe in EFT.
CB: Even though I do not entirely believe in EFT.
UA: Even though I do not entirely believe in EFT.
AFT: Even though I do not entirely believe in EFT.
ToH: Even though I do not entirely believe in EFT.

Round 5

EB: I choose to learn it with an open mind and try it.
SE: I choose to learn it with an open mind and try it.
UE: I choose to learn it with an open mind and try it.
UN: I choose to learn it with an open mind and try it.
CH: I choose to learn it with an open mind and try it.
CB: I choose to learn it with an open mind and try it.
UA: I choose to learn it with an open mind and try it.
AFT: I choose to learn it with an open mind and try it.
ToH: I choose to learn it with an open mind and try it.

Round 6

EB: Even though I do not entirely believe in EFT.

SE: I choose to learn it with an open mind and try it.

UE: Even though I do not entirely believe in EFT.

UN: I choose to learn it with an open mind and try it.

CH: Even though I do not entirely believe in EFT.

CB: I choose to learn it with an open mind and try it.

UA: Even though I do not entirely believe in EFT.

AFT: I choose to learn it with an open mind and try it.

AFT: Even though I do not entirely believe in EFT.

ToH: I choose to learn it with an open mind and try it.

Relax dear, take a couple of deep breaths and calm down. Sip some water. Tell me about your first tapping experience. I wish we could have a 2-way conversation about your first EFT experience. I hope you are feeling calmer. Assess your SUDS score now. Did it surprise you? You may have experienced a significant change or a small change. Even if you haven't witnessed the desired change, please do not be disappointed dear. I am here with you. It is just that you may require some more practice.

I am delighted that you started with EFT and Hearty Congratulations on completing your first tapping experience! (If this was your first) We have plenty of tapping work in this book waiting to **Transform and Lighten you Up!**

I Love & Accept Myself

Part 2

Lighten Your Emotions

Chapter 3

Reducing the Frustration & Anger

Losing weight could be challenging. Especially when you have gained weight after losing it. Your level of motivation, support from family, lifestyle, willpower, and commitment towards your goals all matter. You must not feel burdened and stressed towards losing weight rather feel light and joyful. However, joy can't exist where there are Sadness, Guilt, Anger related emotions. To create more joy and ease, let us identify and shift the unhealthy emotion about how we feel.

So how do you truly feel about losing weight?
Can you name that thought or the emotion that shows up about weight loss? What is it?

Failure?	Embarrassed?	Ashamed?
Guilty?	Angry?	Hopeless?
Fearful?	Sad?	Numb?
Frustrated?	Irritated?	Rejected?
Doubting?	Pressurised?	Stressed & Overwhelmed?

Do these feelings help you to pursue your weight loss goal or does it drain your energy?

As step one, tune into this emotion (the one that you identified) and do 2 rounds of tapping on *This Emotion* or *This Anger* (If it is Anger) to start lowering the emotional intensity.

Rounds 1

KC: This emotion

EB: This emotion

SE: This emotion

UE: This emotion

UN: This emotion

CH: This emotion

CB: This emotion

UA: This emotion

AFT: This emotion

ToH: This emotion

Rounds 2 – Repeat the tapping saying "This emotion"

Once done, relax dear. Take 3 calming deep breaths to release this emotional intensity. Sip some water. Calm down. Make a note of your SUDS score.

You are off to a Great Start!

In the upcoming section and chapters, we will discuss about common unhealthy emotions and learn to tap into them. So now let us dive into reducing these emotions.

Reducing the Frustration

Frustration can be the biggest roadblock towards reducing weight. You could be frustrated for several reasons such as past failures, current weight, your body, your looks, clothes not fitting in and so on. It is important to release the intensity of this frustration and focus on the actions to lose weight. Slight frustration is okay as it would trigger actions towards weight loss. Tap on the reasons for your frustration and reduce it.

Take three deep breaths, tune into this frustration and start tapping. Make a mental note of your SUDS score.

Round 1

KC: Even though I feel frustrated when I tune into my body, I accept how I feel, and I choose to accept myself

KC: Even though I feel irritated when I look at myself, I accept my feelings, and I choose to accept my body.

KC: Even though I feel angry and frustrated about not achieving my weight goals, I accept myself.

EB: I don't know how I became like this

SE: I should have controlled my eating habits

UE: I should have prioritized my health

UN: This is frustrating

CH: Am angry with me

CB: I lost so much time

UA: <Talk about your frustration & tap>

AFT: <Talk about your frustration & tap>

ToH: It's very overwhelming

Round 2

EB: This frustration

SE: This angry feeling

UE: This feeling like a loser

UN: This Regret

CH: This irritation

CB: I do not like myself

UA: I wasted a lot of time

AFT: <Talk about your frustration & tap>

ToH: <Talk about your frustration & tap>

Round 3

KC: Even though I am so done losing weight, I love and accept myself

KC: Even though I am annoyed, as I keep trying to lose weight, but this weight just refuses to go, I choose to accept myself.

KC: Even though I cannot accept myself with my present weight and body, which is frustrating, I choose to accept myself anyway

EB: I just cannot see myself in the mirror

SE: I cannot see the weighing scale

UE: My confidence is shaken

UN: <Talk about your frustration & tap>

CH: <Talk about your frustration & tap>

CB: I feel so angry and frustrated

UA: <Talk about your frustration & tap>

AFT: <Talk about your frustration & tap>

ToH: <Talk about your frustration & tap>

Round 4

Take a pause, a few calming breaths and assess your SUDS score. If you wish to tap more about this issue, go on and do another round of tapping. If you are happy with your progress then proceed further.

Round 5

EB: Even though I am frustrated about not losing weight

SE: Even though I am frustrated about not losing weight

UE: Even though I am frustrated about not losing weight

UN: Even though I am frustrated about not losing weight

CH: Even though I am frustrated about not losing weight

CB: Even though I am frustrated about not losing weight

UA: Even though I am frustrated about not losing weight

AFT: Even though I am frustrated about not losing weight

ToH: Even though I am frustrated about not losing weight

Round 6

EB: I accept how I feel and chose to let go of this emotion.

SE: I accept how I feel and chose to let go of this emotion.

UE: I accept how I feel and chose to let go of this emotion.

UN: I accept how I feel and chose to let go of this emotion.

CH: I accept how I feel and chose to let go of this emotion.

CB: I accept how I feel and chose to let go of this emotion.

UA: I accept how I feel and chose to let go of this emotion.

AFT: I accept how I feel and chose to let go of this emotion.

ToH: I accept how I feel and chose to let go of this emotion.

Round 7

EB: Even though I am frustrated about not losing weight

SE: I accept how I feel and chose to let go of this emotion.

UE Even though I am frustrated about not losing weight

UN: I accept how I feel and chose to let go of this emotion.

CH: Even though I am frustrated about not losing weight

CB: I accept how I feel and chose to let go of this emotion.

UA: Even though I am frustrated about not losing weight

AFT: I accept how I feel and chose to let go of this emotion.

AFT: Even though I am frustrated about not losing weight

ToH: I accept how I feel and chose to let go of this emotion.

Relax dear. Take 3 calming deep breaths to release the emotional intensity. Sip some water. Calm down. Make a note of your SUDS score. Write down any learnings or action points. If you wish, do a round of gamut procedure else express gratitude and close the session.

Brilliantly Done! Sending You Lots of Love & Strength!

Calming The Anger

Similar to frustration, anger is a very unhealthy emotion if not managed and regulated from time to time. A certain amount of anger is healthy as it triggers corrective actions. However, when this emotion is not managed in the right way, it can create heaviness. You could be feeling angry at yourself for your weight loss issue or you could be having suppressed anger for the events in the past not necessarily about losing weight. It is important to let go of this anger, suppressed or presently active to feel calm and lighten yourself. Think about a recent event that made you angry and tap on it.

Suggestive Set up statement to give you a start

Even though he/she should not have said that I now choose to let go of this anger and forgive him/her

Even though he/she should not have done that, I now choose to let go of this anger and forgive him/her

Even though I should not have said that I now choose to let go of this anger and forgive myself

Tap on all the points with the remainder phrases.

Once your emotional intensity of anger is reduced, try and change the thoughts associated with that specific event. Once you shift those thoughts, the intensity of your anger may further reduce as well.

Notice that angry thoughts usually would have words like *Should Be, Must be, Have to, Ought to* etc. This type of thinking is called demanding. When you replace the Should be with - I prefer or I wish, the intensity of your anger may reduce. I explain more about this thinking in the upcoming chapter. However, try to pin down the thought that made you angry and replace that thought starting with I wish or I prefer and notice the change.

Tap on the new/helpful thought for 1 round. For example
Old Angry Thought – He should not have spoken with me in a harsh tone
 New Helpful Thought – I wish that his tone was polite.

Round 1
KC: I wish that his tone was polite.
EB: I wish that his tone was polite.
SE: I wish that his tone was polite.
UE: I wish that his tone was polite.
UN: I wish that his tone was polite.
CH: I wish that his tone was polite.
CB: I wish that his tone was polite.
UA: I wish that his tone was polite.
AFT: I wish that his tone was polite.
ToH: I wish that his tone was polite.

Relax dear. Take 3 calming deep breaths to release the emotional intensity. Sip some water. Calm down. Make a note of your

SUDS score. Write down any learnings or action points. If you wish, do a round of gamut procedure else express gratitude and close the session.

Awesome Stuff! You are Awesome!

I Love & Accept Myself

Chapter 4

Healing The Guilt & Shame

Healing The Guilt

During the process of weight loss, your behaviours and actions can create a feeling of guilt when you eat that extra portion. When you fail to go to the gym or when you give in to the temptation of chocolate. This guilt keeps you away from taking the right action. As per Wikipedia Guilt is a moral emotion that occurs when a person believes or realizes—accurately or not—that they have compromised their standards of conduct or have violated universal moral standards and bear significant responsibility for that violation. Guilt is closely related to the concept of remorse, regret, as well as shame. Guilt is an important factor in perpetuating obsessive-compulsive disorder symptoms as well.

Here is the tapping script to release or reduce the guilt emotion. Take 3 deep breaths, tune in and start tapping.

Round 1

KC: Even though I feel guilty about my poor eating habits which do not help me lose weight, I choose to love and accept myself.

KC: Even though I feel guilty about not controlling my food habits, I accept myself.

KC: Even though I feel guilty about not putting in the effort to lose weight, I choose to accept myself completely.

EB: I cannot follow a good diet plan.

SE: I am unable to control my food cravings.

UE: I binge eat.

UN: I eat a lot of junk food.

CH: There is no discipline in my life.

CB: I do not exercise consistently.

UA: I cannot stop myself from eating those extra portions.

AFT: <Talk about your guilt & tap>

ToH: This guilt of not losing weight.

Round 2

EB: I always feel guilty after I binge

SE: This guilt is bothering me

UE: I know I should control my food cravings

UN: I know I should focus on my weight loss

CH: I am not consistent

CB: This guilt of eating everything I see without any control

AFT: <Talk about your guilt & tap>

ToH: This guilt

Round 3

KC: Even though I feel guilty about my food habits, I accept myself entirely

KC: Even though I am guilty of not consistently working out, I choose to love and accept myself

KC: Even though this guilt is bothersome, I allow myself to heal and let go of this emotion

Tap on all the points and say what naturally comes to you

EB: <Talk about your guilt & tap>

SE: <Talk about your guilt & tap>

UE: <Talk about your guilt & tap>

UN: <Talk about your guilt & tap>

CH: <Talk about your guilt & tap>

CB: <Talk about your guilt & tap>

UA: <Talk about your guilt & tap>

AFT: <Talk about your guilt & tap>

ToH: <Talk about your guilt & tap>

Round 4

Take a pause, a few calming breaths and assess your SUDS score. If you wish to tap more about this issue, go on and do another round of tapping. If you are happy with your progress then proceed further.

Round 5

EB: Even though I feel guilty.

SE: Even though I feel guilty.

UE: Even though I feel guilty.

UN: Even though I feel guilty.

CH: Even though I feel guilty.

CB: Even though I feel guilty.

UA: Even though I feel guilty.

AFT: Even though I feel guilty.

ToH: Even though I feel guilty.

Round 6

EB: I accept myself and chose to release this emotion

SE: I accept myself and chose to release this emotion

UE: I accept myself and chose to release this emotion

UN: I accept myself and chose to release this emotion

CH: I accept myself and chose to release this emotion

CB: I accept myself and chose to release this emotion

UA: I accept myself and chose to release this emotion

AFT: I accept myself and chose to release this emotion

ToH: I accept myself and chose to release this emotion

Round 7

EB: Even though I feel guilty.

SE: I accept myself and chose to release this emotion

UE: Even though I feel guilty.

UN: I accept myself and chose to release this emotion

CH: Even though I feel guilty.

CB: I accept myself and chose to release this emotion

UA: Even though I feel guilty.

AFT: I accept myself and chose to release this emotion

AFT: Even though I feel guilty.

ToH: I accept myself and chose to release this emotion

Relax dear. Take 3 calming deep breaths to release the emotional intensity. Sip some water. Calm down. Make a note of your SUDS score. Write down any learnings or action points. If you wish, do a round of gamut procedure else express gratitude and close the session.

That's Sensational! Superbly Done, Sending You Love!

Healing the Shame

As per Wikipedia, Shame is an unpleasant self-conscious emotion often associated with negative self-evaluation; motivation to quit; and feelings of pain, exposure, distrust, powerlessness, and worthlessness.

You could have this feeling of shame about your body or weight. It is very important to release this emotion and get into a more neutral or positive state about yourself. If the intensity of this emotion is very high, you may want to talk to your therapist. Tune into this emotion of shame and start tapping as below

Round 1

KC: This emotion

KC: This emotion

KC: This emotion

EB: This emotion

SE: This emotion

UE: This emotion

UN: This emotion

CH: This emotion

CB: This emotion

UA: This emotion

ToH: This emotion

Round 2

KC: Even though I feel ashamed to look in the mirror, I choose to deeply accept myself.

KC: Even though I feel bad when I look at the weighing scale, I choose to completely accept myself.

KC: Even though I try to hide my body by wearing loose clothes, I choose to love and accept myself.

EB: I am ashamed of the way I have become

SE: This shame

UE: <Talk about this issue >

UN: It's awkward to step outside my house.

CH: I find it difficult to accept myself.

CB: I do not like my appearance.

AFT: <Talk about this issue >

ToH: I try to hide when I am among people

Round 3

EB: I cannot accept the way I become

SE: I cannot carry myself

UE: I feel so uncomfortable being myself

UN: I just cannot control my eating habits

CH: <Talk about this issue>

CB: It's very embarrassing

AFT: <Talk about this issue >

ToH: I don't know what to do

Round 4

KC: Even though I am ashamed of my weight loss failure, I allow myself to feel okay today.

KC: Even though I am sad and ashamed of not losing weight, I accept myself

KC: Even though I feel ashamed about my body, I accept my body and I choose to love myself

EB: <Talk about this issue >

SE: <Talk about your embarrassment & tap>

UE: I feel so stuck

UN: <Talk about this issue >

CH: I try to avoid getting in the limelight

CB: <Talk about this issue >

UA: It is extremely difficult for me

ToH: <Talk about this issue >

Round 5

Take a pause, a few calming breaths and assess your SUDS score. If you wish to tap more about this issue, go on and do another round of tapping. If you are happy with your progress then proceed further.

Round 6

EB: Even though I feel ashamed about my body & weight.
SE: Even though I feel ashamed about my body & weight.
UE: Even though I feel ashamed about my body & weight
UN: Even though I feel ashamed about my body & weight.
CH: Even though I feel ashamed about my body & weight.
CB: Even though I feel ashamed about my body & weight.
UA: Even though I feel ashamed about my body & weight.
AFT: Even though I feel ashamed about my body & weight.
ToH: Even though I feel ashamed about my body & weight.

Round 7

EB: I accept myself with love
SE: I accept myself with love
UE: I accept myself with love
UN: I accept myself with love
CH: I accept myself with love
CB: I accept myself with love
UA: I accept myself with love
AFT: I accept myself with love
ToH: I accept myself with love

Round 8

EB: Even though I feel ashamed about my body & weight.

SE: I accept myself with love

UE: Even though I feel ashamed about my body & weight.

UN: I accept myself with love

CH: Even though I feel ashamed about my body & weight.

CB: I accept myself with love

UA: Even though I feel ashamed about my body & weight.

AFT: I accept myself with love

AFT: Even though I feel ashamed about my body & weight.

ToH: I accept myself with love

Relax dear. Take 3 calming deep breaths to release the emotional intensity. Sip some water. Calm down. Make a note of your SUDS score. Write down any learnings or action points. If you wish, do a round of gamut procedure else express gratitude and close the session.

That Was Powerful! Sending You Love & Hugs!

I Love & Accept Myself

Chapter 5

Shifting Past Failures & Impatience Energy

Reduce The Weight of Past Failures

Have you tried to lose weight in the past but could not succeed? If yes, tune into that emotion of failure and tap as per the below sequence to overcome the intensity of your past failure. Take three deep breaths, tune into this issue and start tapping:

Round 1

KC: Even though I have no enthusiasm for losing weight, I accept how I feel, and I accept myself.

KC: Even though I have failed to achieve my weight goal, I choose to accept myself completely.

KC: Even though I consider losing weight a big challenge, I accept and love myself.

EB: I have tried to lose weight.

SE: It comes back.

UE: I have failed many times.

UN: It is not easy to lose weight.

CH: I feel low on my energy levels.

CB: I am not sure if I fully believe that I can lose weight.

UA: I lack enthusiasm.

AFT: <Talk about this issue>

ToH: It's too difficult now.

Round 2

EB: I have become sluggish.

SE: There is no excitement left in me to lose weight.

UE: It does not matter whether I lose weight or I don't.

UN: It is okay to be the way I am.

CH: Past failures have been weighing me down.

CB: There is no commitment and no determination.

UA: There is no rush or urgency to lose weight.

AFT: <Talk about this issue>

ToH: There is no discipline to lose weight.

Round 3

KC: Even though my past failures have shaken my confidence, I accept how I feel and choose to love and accept myself

KC: Even though I feel hurt and sad by my failures and attempts to lose weight, I accept and love myself

KC: Even though I have zero confidence in losing weight, I choose to love and accept myself and bring in some courage

EB: <Talk about this issue>

SE: <Talk about this issue>

UE: <Talk about this issue>

UN: <Talk about this issue>

CH: <Talk about this issue>

CB: <Talk about this issue>

UA: <Talk about this issue>

AFT: <Talk about this issue>

ToH: <Talk about this issue>

Round 4

Take a pause, a few calming breaths and assess your SUDS score. If you wish to tap more about this issue, go on and do another round of tapping else move forward.

Round 5

Tap on all the points stating the problem statement. Choose one from the options below or create one of your own.

- Even though my past failure weighed me down
- Even though I have failed many times to lose weight
- Even though I am struggling to lose weight due to past events

Round 6

Tap your love & acceptance or choice statement on all points. Choose one from the options below or create one of your own.

- I love and accept myself
- I accept myself and choose to give my best
- I choose to lose weight with renewed energy

Round 7

Tap on the problem and acceptance statement alternatively.

Relax dear. Take 3 calming deep breaths to release the emotional intensity. Sip some water. Calm down. Make a note of your SUDS score. Write down any learnings or action points. If you wish, do a round of gamut procedure else express gratitude and close the session.

Stupendous! Wish You Loads of Success from now on!

Reducing the Impatience Energy

When we take action with impatient energy, those actions can be stressful. If we are continuously asking questions that start with the word "WHEN" in our mind, then we create an emotion of

anxiety, fear, worry, and feeling restless.
This mind chatter continuously says –
When will I become thin?
When am I going to be happy?
When will I finally lose weight?
When will my waist size reduce?
When will I wear new clothes?

It is time to stop asking these questions and create joyful patience to lose weight with tapping.

How much impatient you are to lose weight? Take three deep breaths, tune into this issue and start tapping:

Round 1
KC: This emotion
KC: This emotion
KC: This emotion
EB: This emotion
SE: This emotion
UE: This emotion
UN: This emotion
CH: This emotion
CB: This emotion
UA: This emotion
ToH: This emotion

Round 2
KC: Even though I am impatient to lose weight, I deeply and completely accept myself

KC: Even though I always keep asking myself "When am I going to lose weight" I accept myself

KC: Even though I get anxious when I do not progress with my weight goal, I accept and love myself

EB: I still have a pretty long way to go.

SE: When are things going to fall into place?

UE: This thought makes me anxious.

UN: I need quick solutions.

CH: I always worry about losing weight.

CB: I keep asking when am I going to get rid of my weight

UA: <Talk about your impatience & tap>

AFT: <Talk about your impatience & tap>

ToH: Too much to do and no support

Round 3

EB: Am getting irritated with this need for patience

SE: When will I become thin?

UE: When am I going to be happy?

UN: When will I finally lose weight?

CH: <Talk about this issue>

CB: When will my waist size reduce?

UA: This weight does not go.

AFT: <Talk about this issue >

ToH: It is tough for me to be so patient.

Round 4

KC: Even though my patience is being pushed to its limits, I deeply and completely love and accept myself

KC: Even though I am expecting to have my patience stretched, I deeply and completely love and accept myself

KC: Even though I am back to square 1 with my weight, and it is very frustrating and overwhelming, I accept myself and relax

EB: I want to lose weight quickly.

SE: I have many things to do.

UE: I keep trying different things to lose weight.

UN: <Talk about this issue >

CH: <Talk about this issue >

CB: <Talk about this issue >

UA: <Talk about this issue >

AFT: <Talk about this issue >

ToH: <Talk about this issue >

Round 5

Take a pause, a few calming breaths and assess your SUDS score. If you wish to tap more about this issue, go on and do another round of tapping else move forward.

Round 6

EB: Even though I am impatient

SE: Even though I am impatient

UE: Even though I am impatient

UN: Even though I am impatient

CH: Even though I am impatient

CB: Even though I am impatient

UA: Even though I am impatient

AFT: Even though I am impatient

ToH: Even though I am impatient

Round 7

EB: I now choose to create joyful patience

SE: I now choose to create joyful patience

UE: I now choose to create joyful patience

UN: I now choose to create joyful patience

CH: I now choose to create joyful patience

CB: I now choose to create joyful patience

UA: I now choose to create joyful patience

AFT: I now choose to create joyful patience

ToH: I now choose to create joyful patience

Round 8

EB: Even though I am impatient

SE: I now choose to create joyful patience

UE: Even though I am impatient

UN: I now choose to create joyful patience

CH: Even though I am impatient

CB: I now choose to create joyful patience

UA: Even though I am impatient

AFT: I now choose to create joyful patience

AFT: Even though I am impatient

ToH: I now choose to create joyful patience

Relax dear. Take 3 calming deep breaths to release the emotional intensity. Sip some water. Calm down. Make a note of your SUDS score. Write down any learnings or action points. If you wish, do a round of gamut procedure else express gratitude and close the session.

That was Awesome! Blossom! Sending You Joy & Patience

I Love & Accept Myself

Chapter 6

Accepting Your Body & Features

Accepting Your Body

Accepting your body and accepting yourself is a great way to heal the drama and trauma around weight loss. It creates lightness and joy by releasing the judgements about your physical appearance. Your perception of your physical appearance or body is very important. It defines how you identify Beauty. We often associate physical beauty as a sign of being successful, being smart or setting a high social status. We dream of a leaner image of ourselves. While it is fine to dream of a slim body, it is also important to acknowledge the real beauty within us. Beauty can come in all shapes and sizes. We tend to lose weight faster when we acknowledge the beauty within us. We go into a state where we do not HAVE TO become lean we still CHOOSE TO become lean. The difference is in the emotional state. The HAVE TO state comes from pressure and stress and trying to fit into society's definition of "Beauty" while the CHOOSE TO state comes from a space of love and freedom. Let us free our conscious and subconscious mind from these judgments we have about our body that often drains our energy. Below steps to assess what judgments you have about your body:

Step 1) Close your eyes and place your hands on your heart.

Step 2) Ask yourself - How am I judging my body?

You may get the awareness of your judgments in the form of a word, feeling, sight or sound or you will just know it.

What did you perceive about your body?

"Chubby", "Fat", "Bulky", "Bulging", "Dark", "Fair", "too tall", "Overweight, "or too short"? Once you get this awareness, tap on those specific judgements you are holding onto about your body or yourself. Take three deep breaths, tune into this judgement, make a mental note of your SUDS score and start tapping:

Round 1

KC: Even though I have become (say what showed up for you) fat, I like to accept myself.

KC: Even though my body is out of shape, I accept my body.

KC: Even though I dislike my body, I choose to accept it.

EB: My body is too fat and round.

SE: I do not like myself in this body.

UE: I do not like to see myself in the mirror.

UN: I did not care about my body.

CH: I do not know how I will get fit.

CB: I don't not how will my body get into a better shape.

UA: I am unhappy with my present weight.

AFT: <Talk about this issue>

ToH: I may have given my body much stress.

Round 2

EB: I have become fat and lazy.

SE: My clothes do not fit.

UE: I wear loose clothes to hide my fat.

UN: I feel so ashamed about being fat.

CH: I feel angry and frustrated that I cannot lose weight.

CB: I must lose weight.

UA: I avoid going to public places.

AFT: <Talk about this issue>.
ToH: This is stressful.

Round 3

KC: Even though I feel miserable about my body, I allow myself to relax with self-acceptance

KC: Even though I cannot look into the mirror and the weighing scale scares me, I accept and love myself.

KC: Even though this is so hard, I accept myself.

EB: My body has become big due to my food choices

SE: I should have taken care of my eating habits

UE: I barely do any exercises to stay fit

UN: I just cry and lie in bed

CH: It's difficult to move my body

CB: I am just lost in social media

UA: I haven't taken care of my health

AFT: <Talk about this issue>

ToH: <Talk about this issue>

Round 4

Take a pause, a few calming breaths and assess your SUDS score. If you wish to tap more about this issue, go on and do another round of tapping. If you are happy with your progress then proceed further.

Round 5

Tap on all the points stating the problem statement. Choose one from the options below or create one of your own.

- Even though I have not accepted my body entirely

- Even though it I very difficult to accept my body

- Even though I am struggling with my physical appearance.

Round 6

Tap your love & acceptance or choice statement on all points.
Choose one from the options below or create one of your own.

- I accept myself and accept my body
- I choose to love and accept my body
- I choose to accept my body with love

Round 7

Tap on the problem and acceptance statement alternatively.

Round 8

EB: I now acknowledge the beauty within me
SE: I now acknowledge the beauty within me
UE: I now acknowledge the beauty within me
UN: I now acknowledge the beauty within me
CH: I now acknowledge the beauty within me
CB: I now acknowledge the beauty within me
UA: I now acknowledge the beauty within me
AFT: I now acknowledge the beauty within me
ToH: I now acknowledge the beauty within me

Relax dear. Take 3 calming deep breaths to release the emotional intensity. Sip some water. Calm down. Make a note of your SUDS score. Write down any learnings or action points. If you wish, do a round of gamut procedure else express gratitude and close the session.

Spectacular! That's the Sign a Champion!

Accept Your Body Features

Similarly, you may find it difficult to accept one or more aspects of your body. For example, a bloated stomach or big arms or lean legs etc. It is essential to accept these aspects of our body too.

What judgments do you have towards your stomach, breasts, thighs, butt, and arms?
Are those judgments helping you?
How uncomfortable do you feel when you tune into this issue?

Let us do tapping taking the example that you are not happy with your stomach. If it is any other part of your body, you are not happy with, then tap accordingly. Take three deep breaths, tune into this issue and start tapping:

Round 1

KC: Even though my stomach is too big, I accept myself and my stomach.

KC: Even though I cannot look at myself in the mirror, I choose to accept myself.

KC: Even though I have failed to tone my stomach many times, I deeply and completely accept myself.

EB: I have failed several times to put my tummy inside.

SE: It is still the same.

UE: I am not particularly eager to carry such a huge stomach.

UN: I feel embarrassed by it.

CH: I feel helpless

CB: I do not know whether my stomach will tone in.

UA: It does bother me.

AFT: <Talk about this issue>

ToH: It is stressful.

Round 2

EB: I feel ashamed.

SE: I have stopped going out.

UE: I do not like the way people stare at it

UN: I hate when people comment behind my back

CH: I cannot wear the clothes I like.

CB: I try to hide it

UA: It is not very pleasant.

AFT: <Talk about this issue>

ToH: I feel angry and stressed

Take a pause and 3-4 breaths. Assess your SUDS score and make a mental note of it.

Round 3

KC: Even though I cannot accept this part of me, I choose to accept it with love

KC: Even though I have been unable to do much about my <body part>, I allow myself to relax and accept myself

KC: Even though it is too overwhelming to tap on this, I accept myself entirely.

EB: <Talk about this issue>

SE: <Talk about this issue>

UE: <Talk about this issue>

UN: <Talk about this issue>

CH: <Talk about this issue>

CB: <Talk about this issue>
UA: <Talk about this issue>
AFT: <Talk about this issue>
ToH: <Talk about this issue>

Round 4

Take a pause, a few calming breaths and assess your SUDS score. If you wish to tap more about this issue, go on and do another round of tapping. If you are happy with your progress then proceed further.

Round 5

Tap on all the points stating the problem statement. Choose one from the options below or create one of your own.

- Even though I dislike my stomach.
- Even though I have no control over my stomach
- Even though I have failed so many times to tone my stomach.

Round 6

Tap on all points except KC with the love and acceptance statement. You can choose one from the below if you like it or create one of your own.

- I love myself and my stomach
- I accept myself and choose to love myself
- I accept myself and make peace with my body

Round 7

Tap on the problem and acceptance statement alternatively.

Round 8

EB: I accept my stomach/ (body part) and make peace with it

SE: I accept my stomach/ (body part) and make peace with it

UE: I accept my stomach/ (body part) and make peace with it

UN: I accept my stomach/ (body part) and make peace with it

CH: I accept my stomach/ (body part) and make peace with it

CB: I accept my stomach/ (body part) and make peace with it

UA: I accept my stomach/ (body part) and make peace with it

AFT: I accept my stomach/ (body part) and make peace with it

ToH: I accept my stomach/ (body part) and make peace with it

Relax dear. Take 3 calming deep breaths to release the emotional intensity. Sip some water. Calm down. Make a note of your SUDS score. Write down any learnings or action points. If you wish, do a round of gamut procedure else express gratitude and close the session.

That's Courageous! Sending You More Courage & Love!

I Love & Accept Myself

Chapter 7

Reducing Emotional Eating

Lowering The Binge for Sweet, Savoury & Beverage

Sometimes, it is the food itself, that triggers unhealthy eating behaviours or binge eating.

Which sugary or sweet food do you often binge on that you absolutely cannot resist?
Or is the salt that you need?
The crunch with the food?

Whatever the case maybe you can tap on that specific food or beverage cravings. Sharing some setup statements and reminder phrases for chocolate, chips and coffee. You can tap on that specific food that you wish to lighten the cravings. It is important that you dig deep when you do tapping on your cravings. Try and assess the underlying emotions and events that are creating the cravings.

For example, let us do tapping on our chocolate cravings. I will share this illustration on how you can dig deep into the root cause of your cravings. I am assuming that your craving has some emotional issue that needs a resolution. Take three deep breaths, tune into the chocolate craving and start tapping. Make a note of your SUDS score.

Round 1

KC: Even though I have a high craving for chocolate, I choose to love and accept myself completely.

KC: Even though eating this chocolate is comforting; I choose to deeply and completely love and accept myself.

KC: Even though eating this chocolate releases my stress, I choose to deeply love myself.

EB: I feel delighted & comforted when I eat this chocolate.

SE: It soothes my heart.

UE: I need to eat it every day.

UN: I receive a sense of ease and peace.

CH: It is my go-to stress buster.

CB: I want to eat it, and I cannot stop myself.

UA: I feel so much at ease, and my stress level goes down.

AFT: It helps me overcome my emotions.

ToH: I need it the most.

Round 2

Do another round of tapping

Round 3

Now try to identify the emotion behind the chocolate craving.

Is it the sadness that you are filling up by eating this chocolate?

Is it anxiety?

Is it the lack of control?

Is it fear?

Once you identify the emotion then tap on that specific emotion in subsequent rounds. There could be multiple emotions that could create this chocolate craving. Identify the underlying emotion by asking questions:

What emotions are creating this craving?

What emotions I am unable to express?

What emotions hide behind this craving?

If I do not eat this chocolate, then what emotion I will have to experience?

Once you have identified the emotion then say out loud that emotion and tap it out. For example, if it is sadness then say:

KC: This sadness

EB: This sadness

SE: This sadness

UE: This sadness

UN: This sadness

CH: This sadness

CB: This sadness

UA: This sadness

AFT: This sadness

ToH: This sadness

Round 4

Once you have tapped out the emotion, ask what events are creating this sadness. Who is associated with this sadness? For example, you went for a job interview but got rejected. This was communicated to you over a phone call that you have been rejected for the job. Then tap on this event. You can choose to say out loud that specific event that is creating this sadness. For example, you could say – *This rejection or this job or this interview.*

KC: This rejection

EB: This rejection

SE: This rejection

UE: This rejection

UN: This rejection

CH: This interview

CB: This rejection

UA: This interview

AFT: This rejection
ToH: This rejection

Round 5

Once you have tapped on this, assess the need to have the chocolate and see if the intensity has reduced. If it has not reduced then try to get to the bottom by asking more questions. In this case, you could be worried about getting a new job. This worry could create anxious feelings. So once again tap on anxiety or you can do a normal tapping round as well.

KC: Even though I am feeling very anxious, I love and accept myself
KC: Even though am unable to relax, I choose to relax now
KC: Even though I am worried, I accept myself
EB: This worry and anxiety
SE: This worry and anxiety
UE: This worry and anxiety
UN: This worry and anxiety
CH: This worry and anxiety
CB: This worry and anxiety
UA: This worry and anxiety
AFT: This worry and anxiety
ToH: This worry and anxiety

Once you have tapped into this aspect, you may notice that your chocolate craving would have reduced drastically. Once you are calm, restart yourself, and start applying aggressively for jobs. Call up your friends and ask for references. Start taking action.

This is the magic of tapping. A chocolate craving was covered in sadness and anxious feelings. Once these emotions and events are tapped, the need to eat chocolate reduces significantly. This is an example of how you can reduce binge eating and cravings.

Similarly, tap on other cravings and try to get to the bottom of the issue. I am sharing a few set-up statements to give you a start. Go on and become lighten and release those cravings.

Set Up & Reminder Phrases for Potato Chips

KC: Even though I have this intense craving to eat these chips, I allow myself to relax.

KC: Even though I must have these chips, I accept myself and choose to relax.

KC: Even though eating these potato chips makes me feel happy and comforted, I choose to accept myself.

EB: This intense craving for chips.

SE: I can taste them now.

UE: The joy of eating them when they are crispy.

UN: It is yummy.

CH: Their saltiness creates a great flavour.

CB: They are my biggest stress busters.

UA: I feel so satisfied when I eat them.

AFT: I cannot control it.

ToH: I need it the most.

Set Up & Reminder Phrases for Coffee

KC: Even though I have this craving for coffee, I deeply and genuinely love and accept myself.

KC: Even though I cannot live without coffee, I accept how I feel and choose to relax now.

KC: Even though I need many cups of coffee every day to keep up with my schedule, I deeply and completely accept myself.

EB: Drinking this coffee makes my nerves calm.

SE: I would get a headache if I do not drink this coffee.

UE: I look forward to drinking coffee each time I take a break

UN: It gives me so much peace and ease.

CH: I need it first thing in the morning.

CB: It has become a basic necessity for me.

UA: I cannot reduce it. I need it.

IF: It gives me a soothing and comforting feeling.

AFT: Consuming coffee is a ritual for me.

ToH: I am uncomfortable even with the thought of reducing coffee.

You Are a RockStar! Way to Go. Congratulations

Release the Need to Eat Food When Stressed

When you are stressed, you could use food as a distraction to calm yourself. Sometimes it is fine. However, if it becomes a habit, then it is important to release it. Identify which emotion leads to this behaviour of binge eating. Do you eat when anxious or sad? Take three deep breaths, tune in & start tapping:

Round 1

KC: Even though I eat to feel comfort during stressful situations, I accept how I feel and choose to relax now.

KC: Even though food relaxes me when I am anxious, I accept and love myself

KC: Even though I eat to avoid being stressed, I deeply and completely love and accept myself.

EB: This anxiety.

SE: It bothers me.

UE: I feel stressed.

UN: This stress.

CH: I feel so low.

CB: It drains my energy.

UA: I need a solution.

AFT: <Talk about this issue>

ToH: I want to resolve this.

Round 2

EB: This food gives me comfort.

SE: My mind receives some relaxation.

UE: I feel slightly better.

UN: I feel some relief with this food.

CH: <Talk about this issue>

CB: I temporarily get into a peaceful state.

UA: I know I should stop this.

AFT: <Talk about this issue>

ToH: I know I should not eat when I am stressed or anxious

Round 3

KC: Even though I am usually stressed and anxious and I do not know how to channel them, I accept how I feel.

KC: Even though I eat when I cannot control the situation, I accept myself and choose to work on this aspect.

KC: Even though I do emotional eating, I accept myself.

EB: <Talk about this issue>

SE: <Talk about this issue>

UE: <Talk about this issue>

UN: <Talk about this issue>

CH: <Talk about this issue>

CB: <Talk about this issue>

UA: <Talk about this issue>

AFT: <Talk about this issue>

ToH: <Talk about this issue>

Round 4

Take a pause, a few calming breaths and assess your SUDS score. If you wish to tap more about this issue, go on and do another round of tapping. If you are happy with your progress then proceed further.

Round 5

Tap your problem statement on all points. For example, even though I eat when I am stressed/anxious/sad.

Round 6

Tap your love & acceptance or choice statement on all points. For example, I choose to release this pattern now or I choose to release this emotion in better ways

Round 7

Tap on the problem and acceptance statement alternatively.

Relax dear. Take 3 calming deep breaths to release the emotional intensity. Sip some water. Calm down. Make a note of your

SUDS score. Write down any learnings or action points. If you wish, do a round of gamut procedure else express gratitude and close the session.

That's a Breakthrough! Congratulations!

Reduce the Cravings When You Sense/Smell Food
The trigger to do food can come when you smell it or see it. To reduce this craving and gain more control when you sense food, below is the suggested tapping script. Tune in, take 3 deep breaths and start tapping.

Round 1
KC: Even though I have no control over food when I smell it, I deeply and completely accept myself.
KC: Even though I cannot resist my food craving when I see it, I choose to love and accept myself profoundly.
KC: Even though I get this intense need to eat when I see or smell my favourite food, I choose to eat consciously
EB: I cannot control my desire when I see or smell food.
SE: It is tempting.
UE: I see the ice cream commercial and get tempted to eat.
UN: I already feel the taste in my mouth.
CH: It's so yummy
CB: My feelings take over me.
UA: My mind makes these decisions.
AFT: I feel so happy and content when I eat it.
ToH: It happens so suddenly.

Round 2

EB: I cannot control it.

SE: I must eat it.

UE: I cannot say no to junk food.

UN: I feel so satisfied when I eat it

CH: I am so content

CB: It all happens so quickly

UA: I lose control

AFT: I don't know what to do about it

ToH: I smell and the sight is irresistible

Round 3

KC: Even though I feel guilty about my food habits, I accept myself entirely

KC: Even though I cannot control myself in those tempting moments, I allow myself to relax

KC: Even though this has been my pattern, I choose to change it with self-acceptance.

EB: <Talk about this issue>

SE: <Talk about this issue>

UE: <Talk about this issue>

UN: <Talk about this issue>

CH: <Talk about this issue>

CB: <Talk about this issue>

UA: <Talk about this issue>

AFT: <Talk about this issue>

ToH: <Talk about this issue>

Round 4

Take a pause, a few calming breaths and assess your SUDS

score. If you wish to tap more about this issue, go on and do another round of tapping. If you are happy with your progress then proceed further.

Round 5

Tap your problem statement on all points. For example, even though I had less self-control over these temptations.

Round 6

Tap your love & acceptance or choice statement on all points. For example, I deeply and entirely love and accept myself.

Round 7

Tap on the problem and acceptance statement alternatively.

Relax dear. Take 3 calming deep breaths to release the emotional intensity. Sip some water. Calm down. Make a note of your SUDS score. Write down any learnings or action points. If you wish, do a round of gamut procedure else express gratitude and close the session.

That's Heart-Warming! Majestic!

Reduce Overeating

When you do food, you become so engrossed in it that you just don't know when to stop eating. Especially when it is your favourite cuisine. Here is a tapping script to help you become more mindful of when to stop eating

Round 1

KC: Even though I know when to stop eating, I deeply and completely accept myself.

KC: Even though I cannot resist my food craving and stop only when the plate is empty and not when I am full, I choose to be more mindful of this pattern

KC: Even though I just don't know when to stop eating and end up overeating, I choose to become more mindful of when to stop.

EB: I cannot control myself when I am eating food

SE: I just don't understand when I should stop

UE: My brain just does not accept that I am full

UN: It is hard for me to stop eating

CH: This overeating has now become a habit.

CB: I hate me when I overeat

UA: I know I should stop but I just cannot stop.

AFT: I feel so engrossed when I eat I forget everything

ToH: It happens so subconsciously.

Round 2

EB: I just cannot stop eating

SE: I eat everything on the plate even if I know I am full

UE: I want to stop at a point when I am full but I cannot

UN: I don't know when I am full

CH: It is hard for me to understand and take action to stop myself

CB: I end up overeating most of the time.

UA: The food takes over me

AFT: I wish to stop this pattern

ToH: I know it is not good for my health

Round 3

Take a pause, a few calming breaths and assess your SUDS score. If you wish to tap more about this issue, go on and do another round of tapping. If you are happy with your progress then proceed further.

Round 5

Tap your problem statement on all points. For example, even though I don't know when to stop myself and end up overeating

Round 6

Tap your love & acceptance or choice statement on all points. For example, I choose to be mindful of when to stop going forward

Round 7

Tap on the problem and acceptance statement alternatively.

Relax dear. Take 3 calming deep breaths to release the emotional intensity. Sip some water. Calm down. Make a note of your SUDS score. Write down any learnings or action points. If you wish, do a round of gamut procedure else express gratitude and close the session.

That was Genius! Phew!

I Love & Accept Myself

Part 3

Lighten Your Thinking

Chapter 8

Shifting The Cognitive Distortions

If I tell you that 1 + 1 = 3. Would you believe it? Am sure you would not. So how did 1+1 become 3 in my view? I did not make a calculation mistake. I made a thinking mistake. Similarly, we can make such thinking mistakes when it comes to weight loss. In my book Calm The Chaotic Mind I talk about 11 such thinking mistakes that create unhealthy emotions. There are some thinking mistakes when it comes to losing weight that creates procrastination tendencies and slows down your progress. It is important to identify these unhelpful thoughts (cognitive distortions) and correct them with helpful ones.

Let us, deep dive, into these thinking distortions and understand their impact and how we can correct them.

Black & White Thinking Distortion

The all-or-nothing or Black and White is extreme thinking. Either This or That is the usual thinking pattern. You either love someone entirely or hate them completely. You aim to become extremely successful or you consider yourself a complete disaster, you either work with 100% commitment or don't work at all. For example, you have started going to the gym and following a good diet to lose weight. However, you cave into the temptation of a cookie. Since your thinking is Black and White, you think that your diet has anyway gone for a toss, and you eat the entire box of cookies or plenty of them. This gets you back to square 1.

Some of the Black and White Thinking examples and their impact are as below:

B&W Thinking: I will give my 100% towards weight loss or not start at all
Impact: It delays your start. Creates procrastination tendencies.

B&W Thinking: Since I am late to go the gym and I cannot work out the full 60 minutes, I will skip going today
Impact: It keeps you away from achieving small success

B&W Thinking: I woke up late, I will start my yoga tomorrow
Impact: It delays your start.

B&W Thinking: As I controlled eating cake for 30 days, today I am going to eat everything
Impact: It takes you back towards gaining weight

B&W Thinking: I did not drink enough water since morning, what is the point in having water now as it's the end of the day
Impact: It ignores the contribution of innumerable small tasks that creates large success

B&W Thinking: I will start my diet only when I consult the best dietician.
Impact: Delay in actions.

B&W Thinking: Either I look the best at the party or don't show up there.
Impact: You eventually don't show up and miss out on the fun aspects

The black-and-white thinking does not allow any scope of midway solutions or grey areas. It is important that you identify such thinking patterns and catch hold of yourself when you think this way. You are a human and bound to make mistakes.

To overcome this thinking, ask yourself questions such as:

- Am I thinking in the extreme?
- Do I see any all-or-nothing thought pattern?
- Are there any grey areas that I can consider?

I would highly recommend that you use the above questions for a week and keep focusing to spot any black-and-white thinking errors. Once you identify this cognitive distortion, apply the Golden Rule of

Something Is Better Than Nothing

Apply this rule by asking yourself **Can I still do something about it?** When you ask this question, you create awareness to do something. You become okay with achieving small tasks. You become ready to get started. No matter how slow the start is or how small the task towards your weight loss is, the important thing is you start doing it. Below are some of the examples you can change your B&W thinking to more helpful thinking.

B&W Thinking: I will give my 100% towards weight loss or not start at all

Helpful Thinking: It is okay if I cannot give 100%. Let me start with 20% today. I could become better and reach my 100% soon.

B&W Thinking: Since I am late to go the gym and I cannot work out the full 60 minutes, I will skip going today

Helpful Thinking: I can still go to the gym and work out for 15 minutes.

B&W Thinking: I woke up late. I will start my yoga tomorrow
Helpful Thinking: I woke up very late and cannot complete all the exercises. Let me start with basic breathing.

B&W Thinking: As I controlled eating cake for 30 days, today I am going to eat everything
Helpful Thinking: I am happy I did not eat the cake for 30 days. I will eat consciously and enjoy it.

B&W Thinking: I did not drink enough water since morning, what is the point in having water now as it's the end of the day?
Helpful Thinking: I could still drink a glass of water and end my day on a good note.

B&W Thinking: I will start my diet only when I consult the best dietician.
Helpful Thinking: I will get started with small things that I already know and consult a dietician.

B&W Thinking: Either I look the best at the party or don't show up there.
Helpful Thinking: I may not look my best now and that's okay. I choose to show up for the party as I do not want to miss out.

Feeling the Lightness With This Shift in Thinking?

Labelling Thinking Distortion

In this thinking distortion, you assign a negative label to yourself. It is a thinking error that could originate from a single adverse event. It takes the form of "Because I did X, I am Y", Labels such as failure, good for nothing, loser, hopeless, and irresponsible are some of them you may label yourself. Here are some examples of how labels get created and how they can be uncreated.

- Because I did not lose any weight last month, I am a failure.
- Because I missed going out for my walk for 2 days, I am irresponsible towards my health and fitness
- Because I gave into the chocolate craving, I am good for nothing.
- Because I could not finish the race, I am a loser
- Because I forgot to wish my mother on her birthday, I am a bad daughter

Assigning yourself labels has repercussions. These labels drain your energy and create unhealthy emotions which further slows down your progress. Let me share a couple of examples.

Label: I did not lose any weight last month ***I am a failure.***
If you consider yourself a failure, you stop giving your 100% not just towards your health, but also to other aspects of your life – be it relationships, work, career or business. Not giving your 100% to other areas of your life, you start noticing the impact in many ways. This re-validates that you are a failure. You start feeling angry, sad or guilty about this aspect.

Label: Because I missed going out for my walk for 2 days, ***I am irresponsible***

The fact that you have labelled yourself as irresponsible, any mistake that you commit gets magnified in the pretext of you not being responsible. This magnification of mistakes, makes you feel guilty and like a failure. If you forget your keys at home, you once again think you are irresponsible. You get the validation and this further makes you upset.

So, every label you assign yourself creates unhealthy emotions that further impact other areas of your life too. It is so important to drop these labels. To uncreate these labels, ask yourself

So What?

- So what if I did not lose weight last month, it does not make me a failure.
- So what if I missed going out for walks, it does not make me irresponsible.
- So what, I gave into the chocolate craving, it does not mean that I am good for nothing.
- So what, I did not finish the race, I will finish it next time. It does not make me a loser. I at least tried
- So what, I forgot to wish my mother this year, I have always celebrated her birthday and I care for her. Not wishing my mother on her birthday does not make me a bad daughter.

The more labels you drop, the lighter you will feel and create more ease and peace in your life and to achieve your goals.

Demanding Thinking Error

You think words – *Should have, should be, he should, I should, I must, he must, need, ought, got to*. This type of thinking implies placing a demand on yourself or the people around you. Some examples of this thinking error are:

- *I must always be perfect*
- *I should never be anxious*
- *I should always be in perfect shape*
- *People should respect me*
- *She should not have said that*
- *I should not have eaten that cake*
- *People should notice me*

Ask yourself if you are thinking in words like - 'should', 'must', 'ought', and 'have to' to make rigid rules about yourself. If you are thinking like this about yourself, then you are implying demands or creating pressure on yourself.

Does thinking like this help you? It is important that you change this demanding thinking to helpful thinking by replacing the *Should be* and the *Must be* by *I wish* or *I prefer*. Examples are below

Demanding: I must always be perfect
Helpful Thinking: I wish I am perfect; however, I am okay if I am not.

Demanding: People should respect me
Helpful Thinking: I wish people respect me. However, not all of

them will and I am fine if they don't too.

Demanding: I should never be anxious
Helpful Thinking: I prefer not to be anxious, however, if am, will take the corrective steps

Demanding: I should always be in perfect shape
Helpful Thinking: I prefer to be in great shape however not being in perfect shape does not impact me

Demanding: I should also always weigh under "X" pounds
Helpful Thinking: I prefer to weigh within "X" pounds however in case I exceed, I will work towards reducing my weight.

Demanding: I should not have eaten that cake
Helpful Thinking: I wish I did not eat that cake. Henceforth I will be more mindful of what I eat

Demanding: People should notice me
Helpful Thinking: It would be nice if people notice me. However, I am okay even if no one does.

Feel the Calmness?

Low Tolerance to Frustration or Boredom

Some people cannot tolerate frustration or boredom. They are likely to assume that something challenging to endure is intolerable. This thinking error magnifies the discomfort in achieving goals. One may tend to quit or procrastinate the task, thinking that it is too dull or frustrating. Also, they underestimate the ability to cope with discomfort. For your weight loss goal, you want to lose weight and start walking on the treadmill. You do it for 3-4 days, and then you get bored. You then decide to walk early morning instead. You experience discomfort waking up early morning and then decide not to pursue your weight loss goal. The boredom to walk on the treadmill and the discomfort of waking up early morning resulted to quit your weight loss goal. Most of the time, things are not served on your platter to enjoy. You have got to put in the hard work to achieve something. Working out on your biceps and triceps can be boring or frustrating when you do not see noticeable results however these activities are important. The Activity-Result Conversion or the output from the activity is not always immediate. It takes time. It takes doing. It gets boring and frustrating, yet it is needed. Learn to do boring things. How? Use a simple self-declaration as below: While you are working on your boring yet important activity, declare to yourself

I Choose to live in my Heart Space

Living in your heart space, there is freedom and lightness. Next time when you do anything boring, try this technique and see the shifts in your being. You need not use this tool only for boring tasks you can use it for tasks that you are supposed to do but do not like to do. Tedious jobs in the office, cleaning the vegetables, washing the utensils, folding clothes etc.

Learn to distinguish between things becoming Difficult Vs Unbearable and Impossible Vs Intolerable. Push yourself to do the tasks even if they give you discomfort in the short term, as they are likely to provide you with results /comfort/ contentment/ happiness in the long term. Am sharing some examples for more clarity and understanding as below:

- Waking up early morning for your walks/run/gym could be difficult but not impossible
- Running on the treadmill can be boring but not unbearable
- Controlling your craving can be frustrating but not intolerable
- Accepting and loving yourself unconditionally can be difficult but not impossible
- Saying No to a friend who is forcing you to eat junk food can be difficult but not heartbreaking

I hope you are with me!

Maximization

It is also called Catastrophizing, and to describe it is making a mountain out of a molehill. We take a minor adverse event and blow it out of proportion by imagining all sorts of disasters resulting from that one single event. You assume the worst-case scenario and jump to the worst possible conclusion. Assuming an accident for late arrival and a break-up for a minor argument are all examples of catastrophic thinking. People with this thinking error think such as:

- As he has not reached home yet, something terrible must have happened to him
- My nose is so big that no one will love me.
- You stand on the weighing scale and your weight shows a fraction high. You maximize this event and think about it the entire day and ruin your day
- You go to a party and a friend asks, "Hey have you put on weight?" You tell your friend that you have not. You come back home and see yourself in the mirror to understand if you

have become big. It's okay to check on yourself and your body. However, do not make it a huge event in your mind.

When you make the small things big, by giving undue importance or continuously thinking about them, then you experience unpleasant emotions. Take a moment and identify 2 things in your life that you are giving under important and catastrophising. How do you feel about this? Do you think that these aspects do not deserve so much of your time and attention? Start snapping out of these thinking mistakes by asking yourself questions like-

- Am I catastrophizing this thought?
- Am I blowing this out of proportion?

De-catastrophising things can create tremendous lightness in your being.

Feeling The Sense of Lightness?

I Love & Accept Myself

Chapter 9

Correcting The Inner Voices

You have a conscious mind and a subconscious mind. Your conscious mind says "I want to lose weight" and your subconscious mind may say "It is not safe to lose weight". This is an example where your conscious mind and your subconscious mind are not in harmony. Your conscious voice has a conflicting subconscious voice. Although the "Even Though" set-up statement corrects this polarity, some voices require a correction. Let us understand what are these inner voices and tap into them

Inner Voice of Safety

This inner voice says "I do not feel safe losing weight".

If you do not feel safe losing weight, ask yourself relevant questions to create awareness about this safety issue.

What will happen if I lose weight?

What am I worried about that makes me feel unsafe?

Do I think that others will take advantage of me?

Other people will be jealous of me and thus reject me.

I won't be able to handle the attention and limelight.

Once you created this awareness then tap on it to release the emotional intensity. Below is a suggestive script to shift this inner voice. Take 3 deep breaths, tune in and start tapping.

Round 1

KC: Even though I do not feel safe because of _____ reason, I love and accept myself.

KC: Even though I do not feel safe because of _____ reason, I choose to take steps to feel safe

KC: Even though I do not feel safe because of _____ reason, I accept myself and choose to feel safe

EB: I feel safe

SE: I do not feel safe

UE: I feel safe

UN: I do not feel safe

CH: I feel safe

CB: I do not feel safe

UA: I feel safe

AFT: I do not feel safe

ToH: I feel safe

Tap more rounds till the time this intensity reduces to an acceptable level

Inner Voice of Willingness

This inner voice is "I am not willing to give my best".

Your best would differ from time to time. Factors like your age, your diet plan, your level of energy, and mental, emotional and physical well-being would determine your best. It is your willingness to give your best that matters the most. If your inner voice or the inner language is that you are not willing to give your best, then that can slow down your weight loss progress. It is important to bring in this shift in your willingness. Below is a suggestive script to increase your willingness to give your best.

Take 3 deep breaths, tune in and start tapping.

Round 1

KC: Even though I am not willing to give my 100% to lose weight, I choose to give my 100% anyway

KC: Even though I am not willing to do my best, I will start slowly and pick up and do my best

KC: Even though my subconscious is not willing to give my best, I now choose to align my conscious and subconscious to be willing to give my best

EB: I am not willing to give my best

SE: I am willing to give my best

UE: I am not willing to give my best

UN: I am willing to give my best

CH: I am not willing to give my best

CB: I am willing to give my best

UA: I am not willing to give my best

AFT: I am willing to give my best

AFT: I am not willing to give my best

ToH: I am willing to give my best

Tap more rounds till the time this intensity reduces to an acceptable level

Inner Voice of Possibility

This inner voice is "It is impossible to lose weight" or "I can't lose weight". If subconsciously you think that you can't lose weight despite your conscious efforts, your progress could drastically get impacted. You may not believe in the possibility of losing weight due to various reasons like past failures, or you cannot envision the new you, or you are trying to lose weight for the first time, or you just do not believe that weight loss is your cup of tea. This lack of belief in the possibility of losing weight becomes a big bottleneck. It is important that you shift this inner voice and start believing in the possibility of weight loss.

Take 3 deep breaths, tune into this issue and start tapping. State the reason you do not believe in the possibility of losing weight.

Round 1

KC: Even though I don't think I can ever lose weight because of past failures I deeply and completely love and accept myself

KC: Even though I don't see the possibility of me losing weight because I have never seen myself in a renewed body, I deeply and completely love and accept myself

KC: Even though I don't believe I can ever lose weight because I am not worthy, I deeply and completely love and accept myself

EB: It is impossible to lose weight

SE: I believe that I can lose weight, slowly but surely.

UE: It is impossible to lose weight

UN: I believe that I can lose weight, slowly but surely.

CH: It is impossible to lose weight

CB: I believe that I can lose weight, slowly but surely.

UA: It is impossible to lose weight

AFT: I believe that I can lose weight, slowly but surely.

AFT: It is impossible to lose weight

ToH: I believe that I can lose weight, slowly but surely.

Tap more rounds till the time this intensity reduces to an acceptable level

While most of us focus on How To lose weight, we should first review our Why or the reason to lose weight. Why do you want to lose weight? To become healthier, to wear the old jeans whatever the reason is, note it. The Why should create the drive and the energy to smoothen your weight loss journey.

Was this helpful? I hope YES.

I Love & Accept Myself

Chapter 10

Releasing Other People's Judgements & Beliefs

Accepting Other Peoples' Judgments

Whether you are fat or thin, rich or poor, smart or dumb other people will judge you. There is no place to hide from other people's judgements. What other people think about you, you have no control and no idea. The problem is when you overthink what they are thinking about you. Lighten this overthinking by tapping on it.

Close your eyes and place your hands on your heart, take 3 deep breaths, and tune in to the thought and emotions of others talking about you and judging you.

How do you think others judge or label you and your body? "Chubby", "Fat", "Bulky", "Fatso", "Dark", "Fair", "too tall", "Overweight", or "too short"? Other people will judge you. No matter what you do. It is vital that you release yourself from their judgments and focus on your best interests.

Take three deep breaths, tune into this issue and start tapping:

Round 1

KC: Even though I think other people are judging me as fatso, I choose to love and accept myself and be in allowance of their judgements.

KC: Even though I feel uncomfortable accepting other peoples' judgments about myself, I completely accept myself.

KC: Even though I am not okay with how I feel others would judge me, I deeply and completely love and accept myself.

EB: They think I am fat & lazy

SE: I feel embarrassed.

UE: It is just too scary.

UN: The world out there can be nasty.

CH: I fear that people will make fun of me.

CB: I am just not comfortable with my body.

UA: What if they are talking bad about me?

AFT: <Talk about this>

ToH: It is tough for me to go out.

Round 2

EB: I cannot dress well

SE: People will talk behind my back.

UE: It is unfair.

UN: I am scared to make new friends.

CH: I feel people will not treat me with respect.

CB: I am not comfortable carrying my body the way it is.

UA: It is stressing me out.

AFT: <Talk about this>

ToH: I hate being judged.

Round 3

Take a pause, a few calming breaths and assess your SUDS score. If you wish to tap more about this issue, go on and do another round of tapping. If you are happy with your progress then proceed further.

Round 4

Tap on all the points stating the problem statement. Choose one from the options below or create one of your own.

- Even though I am uncomfortable being judged by others.
- Even though I do not like the way others judge me
- Even though I resist and avoid other people's judgements

Round 5

Tap your love & acceptance or choice statement on all points. Choose one from the options below or create one of your own.

- I choose to be at peace with their judgments and focus on something worthy.
- I choose to think about my goals and aspirations
- I choose to let go of those thoughts as they are not in my control

Round 6

Tap on the problem and acceptance statement alternatively

Relax dear. Take 3 calming deep breaths to release the emotional intensity. Sip some water. Calm down. Make a note of your SUDS score. Write down any learnings or action points. If you wish, do a round of gamut procedure else express gratitude and close the session.

<u>**SCRIPT TESTING RESULTS**</u>

Participants who used the above tapping script showed continuous improvements in their SUDS score as provided in the below table. The names given below are not the real names of the participants.

Dummy Name	At the Start	After Round 3	After Round 4	After Round 6
John	8	4	2	0
Carol	10	8	5	3
Suzy	9	6	4	2
Jane	10	9	7	3

Release The Need to Fit into Other People's Beliefs

We can subconsciously command our bodies not to lose weight due to social pressures and to fit into other peoples' beliefs. We follow other peoples' rules and behaviours, as well as their advice and belief systems Sharing some examples:

- The people who surround you could be overweight, you could subconsciously mirror them to feel one with them. Because subconsciously your lean image does not align with the people around you. Hence you could subconsciously become overweight to feel a part of them.

- Someone may have told you that you look clumsy when you wear light colour clothes. You accepted this viewpoint as a fact. To fit into this advice and not look clumsy, you have always been wearing dark colour clothes. You and your body have felt very uncomfortable wearing dark colour clothes since the time you started following this advice.

- Someone told you that you should skip breakfast and work out 2 hours every day to lose weight. You have been trying to follow their advice; however, your body feels very uncomfortable. What works for someone else may not work for you and vice-versa.

With the above examples, let us do some introspection:
- What advice have you bought from others which are not helping you lose weight?
- Are you mirroring someone else's reality just to fit in?
- What behaviours and actions you have learned from other people that are draining you now?
- What are you doing to copy others or become like them, that is keeping you away from who you really are?

Take 3 deep breaths, tune into the issue which is appropriate for you and start tapping:

Round 1

KC: Even though I unknowingly followed other people's advice, which caused me and my body much stress, I love and accept myself.

KC: Even though I subconsciously tried to fit into other people's reality to feel accepted and loved, I realize now that I don't have to do that anymore, I accept and love myself

KC: Even though I gave my body much trouble, just to fit into the norms and standards set by others, to avoid being out of place and left out, I accept and forgive myself.

EB: I wish I were more aware.

SE: I made mistakes.

UE: I wish I had received more guidance and awareness.

UN: I regret my decisions since I bought their advice.

CH: I could not identify what was beneficial for my health.

CB: I did not know I was buying other people's advice.

UA: I subconsciously adjusted to other people's norms.

AFT: <Talk about this issue>

ToH: I feel sad when I think about those decisions.

Round 2

EB: I wish I could choose better.

SE: So much time has gone and so much effort has been wasted.

UE: I intend to stop this mirroring.

UN: I choose to be mindful from now on.

CH: I wish somebody had made me aware of this aspect.

CB: I could have avoided so much pain.

UA: I hated eating that extra junk food

AFT: <Talk about this issue>

ToH: I should not have taken those decisions.

Round 3

KC: Even though I followed other's people's advice rather than using my awareness, I deeply accept myself

KC: Even though I should not have listened to them, I had this intuition, but I still did what they said, I choose to forgive myself for everything.

KC: Even though I cannot go back and change the past, I choose to focus on my present and create a beautiful future with love and acceptance.

EB: <Talk about this issue>

SE: <Talk about this issue>

UE: <Talk about this issue>

UN: <Talk about this issue>

CH: <Talk about this issue>

CB: <Talk about this issue>

UA: <Talk about this issue>

AFT: <Talk about this issue>

ToH: <Talk about this issue>

Round 4

Take a pause, a few calming breaths and assess your SUDS score. If you wish to tap more about this issue, go on and do another round of tapping. If you are happy with your progress then proceed further.

Round 5

Tap your problem statement on all points. For example, even though I blindly accepted other people's beliefs.

Round 6

Tap your love & acceptance or choice statement on all points. For example, I now choose to forgive myself and forgive them and move on.

Round 7

Tap on the problem and acceptance statement alternatively.

Relax dear. Take 3 calming deep breaths to release the emotional intensity. Sip some water. Calm down. Make a note of your SUDS score. Write down any learnings or action points. If you wish, do a round of gamut procedure else express gratitude and close the session.

That's Magical! Time to Listen to Your Heart!

I Love & Accept Myself

Chapter 11

Creating The Self-Confidence

If you have directly come to this chapter, then please stop. Go back to the chapter on Correcting Cognitive distortions and read from there on. I assume you have done that so let us proceed.

- Were you 100% confident that you will crack your life's first job interview?
- Were you 100% confident that you will pass your life's first math test?
- Were you 100% confident that you will deliver the best speech, your life's first in front of 1000 people?

I believe the answer to the above questions would be a NO for many of us. You must have practised it several times too yet did not feel 100% confident. With weight loss as well. You know how to lose weight. Perhaps many of you did it earlier too. Yet you do not feel confident. Why is that so?

Because you lack the practical experience to accomplish the task that you do for the first time.

Now let us look at the definition of self-confidence in Wikipedia The concept of self-confidence is commonly defined as self-assurance in one's personal judgment, ability, power, etc. One's self-confidence increases as a result of experiences of having satisfactorily completed particular activities. Self-confidence involves a positive belief that in the future, one can generally accomplish what one wishes to do.

With the above explanation, let us understand some of the features or characteristics of self-confidence:

- Self-confidence would generally be lower if the task to be performed is attempted for the first time.
- Once the tasks are accomplished, your self-confidence increases. (gradually or quickly depending on the task)
- The key to increasing your self-confidence is not in the KNOWING but in the DOING.
- The more you DO, the more you may fail, the more you fail, the more you learn to succeed, and the more you learn to succeed, the more you succeed which eventually increases your beliefs and confidence
- Self-confidence increases your belief to accomplish the same tasks (with greater probability) in future based on your learning and experience
- DOINGNESS is the key while the learning evolves.

Now that you understand what self-confidence means, let us review some DOs and DON'Ts that can help us create self-confidence and also help us prevent breaking it.

DOs

1) Do overcome frustration & boredom tolerance. Overcoming this level of tolerance can boost your confidence.
2) Do follow the rule of Something is better than Nothing. It increases your DOINGNESS in baby steps.
3) Do the tasks even if they may give you slight discomfort initially.
4) Gain knowledge about doing the tasks to increase the chances to succeed at them. Ask people to share their experiences.

5) Do correct your inner voices. If your inner voice of safety, possibility and willingness is not corrected, then your weight loss intention may have loopholes. Your actions may be shallow and hasty. It would not help you build your self-confidence

DONT's

1) Don't Label yourself. Labelling yourself as a failure or loser or irresponsible further delays the DOINGNESS and keeps you entangled in unhealthy thoughts & emotions.
2) Don't think in Black & White because it creates procrastination tendencies and delays your start. This delays your DOINGNESS
3) Don't create unhealthy demands on yourself. *I MUST ALWAYS LOOK PERFECT*. When you create such a demand, and during days when you aren't looking your best, what happens? It shakes your confidence and then you go into the negative thought-emotion loop.
4) Don't Maximize. When you see a few pounds have increased on the weighing scale, acknowledge it. Review and understand why it increased. Start DOING activities to bring it down. Don't continuously think about it and spoil your day. If you do, you slowly reduce your self-confidence
5) Don't listen to other people's beliefs & opinions.

Taping on the self-confidence aspect can also help you increase your self-confidence. To help you get a start, below are some creative tapping Set-up statements.

- Even though I lack self-confidence in losing weight, I choose to love and accept myself. I choose to lose weight with confidence

- Even though I haven't figured out, how to lose weight, I choose to believe and trust myself to lose weight

- Even though I have zero confidence to lose weight, I choose to start doing things to regain my confidence

- Even though my confidence today is very low, I acknowledge it and accept myself. I choose to work on it slowly and steadily by accomplishing small tasks.

- Even though my self-confidence is shaken, I accept myself and choose to work on my self-confidence with love.

- Even though I have never lost weight, I choose to bring my A game

Feeling Confident Already? I bet You are.

I Love & Accept Myself

Part 4

Lighten Up Your Heart

Chapter 12

Subsiding the Fears & Pressures

What is the weight of the fears and pressure on yourself?

Would you like to feel lighter by offloading that weight?

This weight comes in the form of fear of failure, the fear of gaining weight once you have lost it, the fear of handling people's questions and comments after you have lost weight, the pressure to succeed, the new identity etc. Let's do tapping into these aspects.

Reducing Fear of Failure

Does this fear of failure leads to procrastination tendencies and does not even help you get started?

Does this fear drain your energy?

Let's diffuse this fear with tapping. Take 3 deep breaths, tune into this fear of failure and start tapping.

Round 1

KC: Even though I am so afraid of failing, I accept how I feel and choose to love and accept myself.

KC: Even though I fear not losing weight at all, I allow myself to relax and accept myself.

KC: Even though I am worried about failure to achieve my goal, I deeply love and accept myself.

EB: I could fail to achieve my goal.

SE: I would feel very sad.

UE: It may shake my confidence.

UN: I cannot imagine myself failing.

CH: I am putting in so much effort

CB: I cannot afford to fail this time.

UA: I fear that if I fail this time, I will never lose weight

AFT: <Tap and say what you feel>

ToH: What if I fail?

Round 2

EB: This fear.

SE: I am worried about not losing weight.

UE: I do not allow myself to fail.

UN: I am afraid to fail.

CH: What if my plan does not workouts?

CB: What if I cannot lose weight?

UA: What if there is a hindrance in my weight loss plan?

AFT: All this stress and pressure

ToH: What if I do not become leaner?

Round 3

KC: Even though I may fail again, I accept myself

KC: Even though am not sure of achieving my weight loss goal, I love and accept myself

KC: Even though I fear not losing weight, I choose to relax now.

EB: <Talk about this issue>

SE: <Talk about this issue>

UE: <Talk about this issue>

UN: <Talk about this issue>

CH: <Talk about this issue>

CB: <Talk about this issue>

UA: <Talk about this issue>

AFT: <Talk about this issue>
ToH: <Talk about this issue>

Round 4

Take a pause, a few calming breaths and assess your SUDS score. If you wish to tap more about this issue, go on and do another round of tapping. If you are happy with your progress then proceed further.

Round 5

Tap on all the points stating the problem statement. Choose one from the options below or create one of your own.

- Even if I fail to lose weight.
- Even though I may not achieve my goal
- Even though I fear I could fail

Round 6

Tap your love & acceptance or choice statement on all points. Choose one from the options below or create one of your own.

- I promise to love and accept myself anyway
- I choose to love and accept myself
- I choose to give my best shot at it

Round 7

Tap on the problem and acceptance statement alternatively.

Relax dear. Take 3 calming deep breaths to release the emotional intensity. Sip some water. Calm down. Make a note of your SUDS score. Write down any learnings or action points. If you wish, do a round of gamut procedure else express gratitude and close the session.

That's Extraordinary! Way to Go!

Reducing Fear of "If I lose weight, I will gain it back."

How much do you fear that once you lose weight, you will gain it back?

Do you feel that maintaining your weight will be a challenge?

Take three deep breaths, tune into this issue and start tapping:

Round 1

KC: Even though I fear that I will gain back the weight I have lost; I choose to love and accept myself.

KC: Even though I fear that I will not maintain my weight, I like to love and accept myself.

KC: Even though I fear gaining weight, I choose to accept myself and allow myself to be at ease.

EB: I am scared. What if I gain back the weight?

SE: I cannot take actions to lose weight.

UE: This fear keeps pulling me down.

UN: Since I will gain weight, I instead do not try

CH: This intense fear of gaining weight.

CB: It is frustrating as it has happened to me earlier.

UA: It keeps on bothering me.

AFT: Am worried that all my efforts will go in vain.

ToH: It does not allow me to give my best.

Round 2

EB: What if I become fat again?

SE: What if I fail to maintain my weight?

UE: All the time and effort would be wasted.

UN: I would be sad if this happens.

CH: I may lose my confidence if I would gain the weight back.

CB: I would feel ashamed.

UA: This is all too stressful.

AFT: <Talk About this issue>

ToH: What would other people think about me?

Round 3

KC: Even Though, <Talk about this issue>

KC: Even Though, <Talk about this issue>

KC: Even Though, <Talk about this issue>

EB: <Talk about this issue>

SE: <Talk about this issue>

UE: <Talk about this issue>

UN: <Talk about this issue>

CH: <Talk about this issue>

CB: <Talk about this issue>

UA: <Talk about this issue>

AFT: <Talk about this issue>

ToH: <Talk about this issue>

Round 4

Take a pause, a few calming breaths and assess your SUDS score. If you wish to tap more about this issue, go on and do another round of tapping. If you are happy with your progress then proceed further.

Round 5

Tap on all the points stating the problem statement. Choose one from the options below or create one of your own.

- Even though I fear gaining weight
- Even though I am afraid of putting on more weight
- Even though I am unsure of maintaining my weight

Round 6

Tap your love & acceptance or choice statement on all points. Choose one from the options below or create one of your own.

- I love and accept myself
- I choose to give my best
- I decide to lose weight with trust & confidence

Round 7

Tap on the problem and acceptance statement alternatively.

Relax dear. Take 3 calming deep breaths to release the emotional intensity. Sip some water. Calm down. Make a note of your SUDS score. Write down any learnings or action points. If you wish, do a round of gamut procedure else express gratitude and close the session.

That's Powerful! More Power To You!

<u>SCRIPT TESTING RESULTS</u>

Participants who used the above tapping script showed continuous improvements in their SUDS score as provided in the below table. The names given below are not the real names of the participants.

Name	At the Start	After Round 3	After Round 5	After the Round 7
Shweta	10	7	4	0
Shilpa	10	9	6	2
Varsha	10	7	5	2
Poonam	8	5	3	1

Reduce the Fear of Success

What would your thoughts, feelings and beliefs be after you have lost weight?

Are you ready and willing to succeed?

How do you feel when you imagine yourself in the new you?

Do you feel uncomfortable?

Would you be able to manage other peoples' reactions and comments?

Do you fear losing weight to avoid the limelight?

Take three deep breaths, tune into this issue and start tapping:

Round 1

KC: Even though I have this fear of self-acceptance after I have lost weight, I love and accept myself.

KC: Even though I am worried about having a complete change in my identity, I choose to love and accept myself.

KC: Even though I am worried about how I will answer people's comments and questions, I choose to accept myself.

EB: Will I be able to identify myself in the new me?

SE: Will other people be able to identify and relate with me?

UE: People would notice the change in me.

UN: They may stare at me.

CH: They may think about what is wrong with me.

CB: I am scared to be in the limelight.

UA: What if I cannot manage the attention?

AFT: <Talk about this issue>

ToH: I am not ready to answer people's questions.

Round 2

EB: People may suddenly see me as weak or ill.

SE: They will enquire with my family about any wellness issues.

UE: Some may be silently jealous of my weight loss.

UN: How will I answer their questions about my health?

CH: I do not know how will others accept the new me.

CB: I am worried that I will lose my friends.

UA: All this pressure and stress

AFT: <Talk about this issue>

ToH: There will be nothing for me to work on later.

Round 3

KC: Even though I am scared about an identity change, I accept this transformation with love.

KC: Even though this would be a big change, I truly love to accept myself and embrace this change

KC: Even though it could be difficult initially, I choose to be confident to accept the new me.

EB: <Talk about this issue>

SE: <Talk about this issue>

UE: <Talk about this issue>

UN: <Talk about this issue>

CH: <Talk about this issue>

CB: <Talk about this issue>

UA: <Talk about this issue>

AFT: <Talk about this issue>

ToH: <Talk about this issue>

Round 4

Take a pause, a few calming breaths and assess your SUDS score. If you wish to tap more about this issue, go on and do another round of tapping. If you are happy with your progress then proceed further.

Round 5

Tap on all the points stating the problem statement. Choose one from the options below or create one of your own.

- Even though I am afraid of having a new identity
- Even though I am not sure how will I handle people's questions and judgements
- Even though I feel this fear of success

Round 6

Tap your love & acceptance or choice statement on all points. Choose one from the options below or create one of your own.

- I choose to embrace this change with love
- I trust myself and welcome this change
- I choose to accept this transformation with love

Round 7

Tap on the problem and acceptance statement alternatively. Once done, take three deep breaths, express gratitude, make a note of your final SUDS score and close the session.

That was Magical! Way to Go!

Release the Pressure of Success

How much pressure do take to achieve your weight goal?

Is this pressure draining you down? If yes, take 3 deep breaths, tune into this pressure and start tapping:

Round 1

KC Even though I take much stress to lose weight, I deeply and completely love and accept myself.

KC Even though I take pressure to lose weight, I accept myself and decide to go easy.

KC: Even though I take much pressure to achieve my goal, I like to relax and be at ease.

EB: I am generally too hard on myself.

SE: I cannot relax.

UE: I got to lose weight anyhow.

UN: I often exert my body.

CH: I don't give myself enough mental breaks and rest.

CB: I cannot relax till I lose significant weight.

UA: The pressure is just so much.

AFT: <Tap and say what you feel>

ToH: All this pressure.

Round 2

EB: I have so much to do.

SE: I have such a long way to go.

UE: I do not allow myself to fail.

UN: There is so much hard work.

CH: It's challenging.

CB: All this pressure and stress

UA: So many expectations from myself and others.

AFT: So much to do and so little time.

ToH: I have told everybody about my weight loss goal, and hence I better achieve it.

Round 3

KC: Even though losing weight is very overwhelming, I love and accept myself

KC: Even though weight loss is extremely challenging, I love and accept myself

KC: Even though this pressure I create is so high, I allow myself to breathe and relax

EB: <Talk about this issue>

SE: <Talk about this issue>

UE: <Talk about this issue>

UN: <Talk about this issue>

CH: <Talk about this issue>

CB: <Talk about this issue>

UA: <Talk about this issue>

AFT: <Talk about this issue>

ToH: <Talk about this issue>

Round 4

Take a pause, a few calming breaths and assess your SUDS score. If you wish to tap more about this issue, go on and do another round of tapping. If you are happy with your progress then proceed further.

Round 5

Tap on all the points stating the problem statement. Choose one from the options below or create one of your own.

- Even if I fail to lose weight.
- Even though I may not achieve my goal
- Even though I expect to lose weight

Round 6

Tap your love & acceptance or choice statement on all points. Choose one from the options below or create one of your own.

- I promise to love and accept myself anyway
- I choose to give my best shot at it
- I choose to lose weight with love and ease

Round 7

Tap on the problem and acceptance statement alternatively.

Relax dear. Take 3 calming deep breaths to release the emotional intensity. Sip some water. Calm down. Make a note of your SUDS score. Write down any learnings or action points. If you wish, do a round of gamut procedure else express gratitude and close the session.

Brilliantly Done! You Will Lose Weight! You Will Shine!

I Love & Accept Myself

Chapter 13

Accepting & Loving Yourself

Unconditional love and self-acceptance go a long way to help you be at peace and grow in life not just lose weight. Here is a simple yet powerful tapping script to love and accept yourself unconditionally. Look at yourself in the mirror, sit in a comfortable position, take 3 deep breaths and start tapping:

Round 1

KC: I accept and love myself unconditionally.
EB: I accept and love myself unconditionally.
SE: I accept and love myself unconditionally.
UE: I accept and love myself unconditionally.
UN: I accept and love myself unconditionally.
CH: I accept and love myself unconditionally.
CB: I accept and love myself unconditionally.
UA: I accept and love myself unconditionally.
AFT: I accept and love myself unconditionally.
ToH: I accept and love myself unconditionally.

Self-Love & Self-Care

Tap a few rounds and raise your self-love quotient. Just tapping and doing nothing does not help. You got to start loving and taking care of yourself.

**Love yourself so much that others
fall in love with your being**

Take care of yourself like you would take care of your child.

Take responsibility for your mental, emotional and physical well-being. Listen to soft music, burn a candle, take a long bath, be with nature, hug a tree, and play with your dog. Call up an old friend and check on him/her.

Be fully present when you take your meal with your family

Do things that bring you joy and make you happy.

Be with people who make you feel loved and are loved too. Let your ultimate goal in life, be living life fully. Being in the present. Enjoying your life, health and relationships.

Celebrate Life!

Self-Acceptance

By now, with tapping, you would have already accepted and made peace with weight loss issues. I'd like you to go one step beyond. Not just about weight issues, but for everything else as well, accept yourself. In life, you will experience the highs and the lows. Sometimes you become thin, sometimes fat. Sometimes you succeed; at times you fail. Sometimes you get lucky, and sometimes luck does not favour you. Life is a series of such events (the good, the bad and the ugly). It is important that when such events are happening to you, then you do not resist them. Accept it, move on and take the required actions.

- Gained 30 pounds? Accept it. Work towards losing weight.
- Lost your wallet. Accept it. Be aware next time
- Living in a small house. Accept it. Plan towards a bigger house and work towards it
- Made a big financial blunder. Accept it. Learn from your mistake. Become wise.

- Clothes not fitting in? Accept it. Lose weight and then wear them or buy new ones.

Not just life events, it is important to accept yourself entirely. The person, who you truly are. Your pros and cons. Your gifts and talents. Your drawbacks. Everything about you, your past, your present, your health, relationships, work, career etc. Using the set-up statements for acceptance can do wonders to create massive peace in your heart. Below are some suggestions on how you can accept your drawbacks or things not working for you to help you get started.

Self-Acceptance Set Up Statements.

You can choose one or create of your own. Keep tapping on one aspect till you feel you have accepted that aspect. You can choose to do entire rounds of tapping as well based on the intensity of the issue.

- Even though I don't love my job, I accept it
- Even though I am not rich, I accept it
- Even though I hate my boss, I accept him/her
- Even though my son does not listen to me, I accept it.
- Even though I am not living my full potential, I accept it.
- Even though I cannot control my anger, I accept it.
- Even though I am having a difficult time in my relationship with X person, I accept it.
- Even though I cannot run fast as I did a few years ago, I accept it.

Once you accept yourself and the aspects that you are not okay with, you create peace in your heart. The major work is done. The next step is working towards those aspects.

For example, simply accepting the fact that you cannot control your anger does not help you or others around you. You got to put in the effort to meet your counsellor, take some anger management training and learn the skill to manage your anger.

Simply accepting that you are not living your full potential won't help. You got to put yourself out there. Explore opportunities. Experiment and try out new things.

Simply accepting your damaged relationship won't help, you got to do what you got to do. Acceptance should be followed by inspired actions. You will learn more about inspired actions in the upcoming chapter.

You are Perfect with your Imperfections!

I Love & Accept Myself

Chapter 14

Forgiveness & Gratitude

The forgiveness prayer can miraculously open things in your universe by healing or clearing various known or unknown blockages. You ask for forgiveness by tapping on all the body points and saying, "I am sorry, please forgive me, thank you, I love you, I forgive myself. Below is what you can tap on.

KC: Dear Body, I am sorry, please forgive me, thank you, I love you, I forgive myself.
EB: Dear Body, I am sorry, please forgive me, thank you, I love you, I forgive myself.
you, I forgive myself.
UA: Dear Body, I am sorry, please forgive me, thank you, I love you, I forgive myself.
And so on...

Relax dear. Take 3 calming deep breaths to release the emotional intensity. Sip some water. Calm down. Write down any learnings or action points.

That's Deep Healing!

Not just with your body, you could do forgiveness wherever you experience unhealthy and heavy emotions. For example, you may not be happy with your relationship with your father due to several events that have happened in the past. You could ask for forgiveness (silently and energetically) and start healing your relationship with your dad. The prayer of forgiveness is beautiful and powerful. It can create a massive shift in your and your dad's level of consciousness. Tune into the emotions you are experiencing with your father and tap from KC point to Top of Head.

Dear Father, I am sorry, please forgive me, thank you, I love you, I forgive myself.

Miracles Happen with Forgiveness.

Being Grateful to Your Body

We all know the power and magic of gratitude. You can tap on the below sequence to express your gratitude towards your body. Sit in front of a mirror, take 3 deep breaths and start tapping as

KC: Dear Body, I Thank You for Everything
EB: Dear Body, I Thank You for Everything
SE: Dear Body, I Thank You for Everything
And so on…

Do more tapping rounds as needed. Once done, keep both your hands on your face. Try to cover your entire face. Be in this moment as much as you like and once again express gratitude towards your body. Take three deep breaths, sip some water and close the session.

Shifting Focus With Gratitude

Sometimes, we could give undue importance to weight loss and neglect other areas of life. We could ignore our gifts and achievements. It is important to have a balanced view towards life. Creating a balance towards your health, relationships, work, career, personal goals etc makes life beautiful. Do a few rounds of gratitude tapping and raise your lightness. You could do gratitude tapping in 2 methods. The first is to tap and express gratitude for everything you have.

Method 1

KC: I am grateful to my spouse for always being around me

EB: I am grateful that I have a good job

SE: Am grateful to live in a lovely home

UE: I express my gratitude for the food I eat

UN: Am glad that I can work from home

CH: I am grateful that I dance so well

CB: I am grateful to have a loving dad/mom/sister/brother.

UA: I am grateful that I have all the amenities to live a comfortable life

AFT: I am grateful to receive support whenever I need

ToH: I am grateful to my body

Method 2

In this method you start saying

Even Though <Talk about your present body & weight issue> and then express your gratitude for something much beyond your weight issue.

KC: Even though I do not have the perfect body, I am grateful to have a loving spouse/parent/son/daughter

EB: Even though I do not have the right shape, I am grateful that I am in the right job

SE: Even though I do not have gym equipment, am grateful that I have a lovely house.

UE: Even though, I cannot resist sweet cravings, I and grateful that there is food on my plate

UN: Even though the gym is too far from my house, am glad that I can work from home and spend some time walking

CH: Even though I do not look in the best of shape, I am grateful that I dance so well

CB: Even though my gym trainer is very strict, am glad that I have one.

UA: Even though my waistline just does not reduce, I am grateful that I have all the amenities to live a comfortable life

AFT: Even though my family does not support me as much in losing weight, I am glad I have a family who supports me in everything else.

ToH: Even though my body needs to be lighter, I am glad that my heart is light and full of compassion.

Decide which method works best for you and accordingly do the gratitude tapping.

Feeling The Magic?

I Love & Accept Myself

Chapter 15

Taking Inspired Actions

This is the last chapter of the book. I assume you have read the book from the beginning and done several rounds of tapping and feeling a lot lighter than before. Am sure the issues that were bothering you earlier have subsided. If it has not, then please go back to the earlier chapters, resolve those issues and then come back to read this chapter.

I assume you have come back after resolving those issues. It is now time to take inspired actions towards losing weight. Am sure many of you would have already started taking physical actions towards losing weight – like going to the gym, eating healthy, walking, reducing binge eating etc. If you haven't then do not be disappointed. Here is a tapping script that can create power in your being and help you take inspired actions:

Round 1

KC: I now tap into my power to take inspired actions

EB: I acknowledge my inner strength and beauty

SE: I choose to take actions with ease and love

UE: I am powerful, lovable and worthy

UN: I am now 100% focused, strong and ready to do what it takes to accomplish all my goal

CH: I am grateful for everything that I have and I progress towards everything I want with clarity and enthusiasm

CB: I keep things simple and focus on my universe

UA: I am a superpower and I know I will achieve my goal

AFT: I take inspired actions from here and now
ToH: My thoughts, feelings and actions are in harmony.

Do more rounds of tapping as you need till the time you feel aligned to take the specific actions that will help you achieve your weight loss goal.

Feeling Super Charged?

Creating a Daily Tapping Routine

Commit yourself to 15 minutes of tapping in the morning (does not have to be immediately after you wake up) and another 5 to 7 minutes at a time in the day when your energy is down or you are feeling stressed/ low or any unhealthy emotions.

Begin your morning by tapping on the issue that is bothering you most. This does not necessarily have to be the weight issue. For example, let us say, you are worried about matters related to finances, then tap 3-4 rounds in the morning about money till you are calm. Once you are more relaxed and at ease, then tap on the specific weight loss issue.

If multiple things are bothering you, then you can also do some generic tapping to start with such as *Everything bothering me now, everything about my work bothering me, everything about my spouse worrying me, my financial situation, everything about my health, all the complaints about my son etc.* All that you have to do is tap on each body point saying out loud what is bothering you. So, to summarize your morning tapping sequence could have general tapping about *everything bothering you,* tapping on the urgent non-weight issue and then tapping on the specific weight loss issue.

That's it. Isn't it Simple?

Joyful Actions

Not all actions to lose weight need to be difficult and involve willpower. Some actions, which I consider joyful are tremendously helping me to shed pounds and I would love to share that. I dance for about 30 to 40 minutes every day. Some days I dance for 60 minutes and some days 20 and some I just do light walking. As each day is different, I acknowledge it and adjust to my schedule while I am maintaining the consistency to move my body.

What joyful activities can you do to move your body?

Playing tennis, swimming, basketball, cycling, running with your dogs, hitting the gym, running on the treadmill? A mix of many activities? Choose what gives you joy and then start moving your body consistently. You can choose different activities each day too. There are no forms and structures when it comes to moving your body. Go with the flow and enjoy each day as it comes.

I also drink lots of water every day. It keeps me hydrated. I eat fruits and healthy foods. What are the healthy foods that can bring joy to you? Identify those foods and start eating. Simple! Identify that 1 thing that gives you immense joy and do it every day. This is nothing to do with weight loss. But this is everything to do to be happy. Playing with your kid, a nap in the afternoon, watching Netflix, playing the piano, reading a book, listening to music, coding, playing cricket? Whatever that activity is, just do it. Everyday! It will supercharge your being.

I also eat my food slowly and consciously. I relish every bite. I make my jaw put more effort. Practice slow and conscious eating. When you eat, look very closely at the colour of the food, notice the texture, and consciously notice what is going on inside your mouth. Feel the morsels of the food you are eating. If you take 15 minutes to have your meal, try to complete your dinner in 25 to 30 minutes. Eat slowly and enjoy your food. If you cannot control that cake craving, use this technique when you eat the cake. Eat slowly and enjoy it thoroughly. Be in the present moment. Be fully engaged in experiencing the taste of the cake. When you do this, you will be surprised that the quantum of cake you ate will be less than what you anticipated. You would receive the same amount of joy by eating a tiny piece of cake. Conscious eating allows your body to receive and enjoy the meal entirely. It also helps your body to slow down and be calmer.

Before you go to sleep, write down what is bothering you on a piece of paper. Write whatever comes to your mind. Acknowledge the worries and stresses by writing them down. Once noted, tell your higher power or divine source or someone you believe in to resolve your issues and concerns, and then go to sleep. Surrender to the higher power everything that is bothering you and then sleep peacefully. Your notes can be as follows.

- *I am worried about getting fired from my job*
- *I am stressed about not losing weight*
- *I am unsure whether my business will do well*
- *Am concerned about the meeting tomorrow*
- *Am worried about money*

It's important that you relax your mind and body before your sleep. Listen to your favourite music or check out the ones related to progressive muscle relaxation to help you relax.

I am now going to share with you an undiscovered secret for losing weight. Wanna know? I bet you want, so here it is…

Inspired Actions with Self Love

That's my undiscovered secret to feeling light and losing weight. In the name of consistency, we could push ourselves too much. It is important to draw a line between consistency and self-love. For example, you decided that you will stop eating cookies for 3 months. You have successfully not eaten a single cookie for 2 months in a row. That's consistency & inspired action. One fine day you meet your friends over coffee and they serve cookies. They all are cherishing the cookies while you are salivating watching them. Don't stop yourself in the name of commitment. A single cookie won't disrupt your weight loss goal. Grab a cookie and enjoy it. I am saying grab A Cookie and not 5 of them. Eat that one cookie with love and happiness. That's Self Love. Let your inspired actions and commitment to lose weight, come from a space of love rather than stress or pressure. When you do this, you create a good balance between your inspired actions that align with your consistency within the space of love and freedom.

Be Consistent to Love Yourself.
Take Inspired Actions Consistently

I Love & Accept Myself

DEDICATION

My Dear, this book is dedicated to you.

I Thank you for reading this book and I truly wish that your effort to implement EFT on your weight issues has created a positive change in you and in your life.

Please do write to me at kunaldudejacoach@gmail.com if you wish to share your feedback about your shifts and transformations. I would be delighted to see your note.

I wish you loads of love and success in all your life's endeavours.

Stay Blessed and Lighten Up!

KD

GRATITUDE AND ACKNOWLEDGEMENTS

I am most grateful to Mr Gary Craig, who invented the Emotional Freedom Technique and my numerous clients; your feedback and progress inspired me to write this book.

I am grateful to my parents, for always showering their blessings and guiding light from heaven above. I express my deep gratitude to my wife for being a great support and to my cute little daughter; both have played a pivotal role by just being there with me in all of my life's ups and downs.

Heartfelt gratitude to my teacher Mr Prasenjit Kamble. The way you have taught me EFT, I could not have asked for a better teacher. Your guidance and techniques helped me create the scripts and test them with some of your students who added their valuable input.

Am grateful to Suzy Woo for always supporting me, Graham Nicholls for sharing in-depth knowledge on EFT, Kain Ramsay for the incredible course on CBT, Center of Excellence & Endorphin, Matthew Barnett for learning NLP, Nitin Soni and Som Batla, Vigneshwari Abraham has inspired me constantly. My batch mates of leadership training programs, Krishan Kakrecha for designing the book cover.

I take the opportunity to thank my incredible family, friends and well-wishers for their continued support – My Family (Gulab, Kirti, Sunita, Karishma, Akshay, Megha, Shantanu, Amita, Vishal, Ranjit, Priya) and my friends – Amit, Swati, Khushi,

Rahul, Kavita, Rushabh, Shweta, Makarand, Niraj, Varsha, Prakruti and all the others who helped me in the past and those who will stand by me in the future.

I have been inspired by reading these books and received some amazing insights. I would highly recommend reading them. I acknowledge the below book's contributions to my life and the motivation to write Lighten Up!

- EFT for Weight Loss – Gary Craig
- The Tapping Solution: A Revolutionary System for Stress-Free Living – Nick Ortner & Mark Hyman
- The EFT manual -Dawson Church
- The Tapping Solution: For Weight Loss & Body Confidence – Jessica Ortner
- The Book of Tapping – Sophie Merle
- Cognitive Behavioural Therapy Workbook for Dummies – Rhena Branch & Rob Willson
- Feeling Good – David D Burns
- Tapping The Healer Within- Roger Callahan
- Calm The Chaotic Mind – Kunal Dudeja

ABOUT ME

Am Kunal Dudeja, better known as KD. By heart, I consider myself a trainer. I believe in empowering and training people with EFT and CBT tools and techniques. I have worked with thousands of souls across the globe through empowering workshops. I conduct online individual consultation sessions with love and simplicity. To know more about me, visit www.kunaldudeja.com.

I also authored the book Calm The Chaotic Mind. A book that helps create peace of mind during life's chaotic situations and more calm for daily stressors.

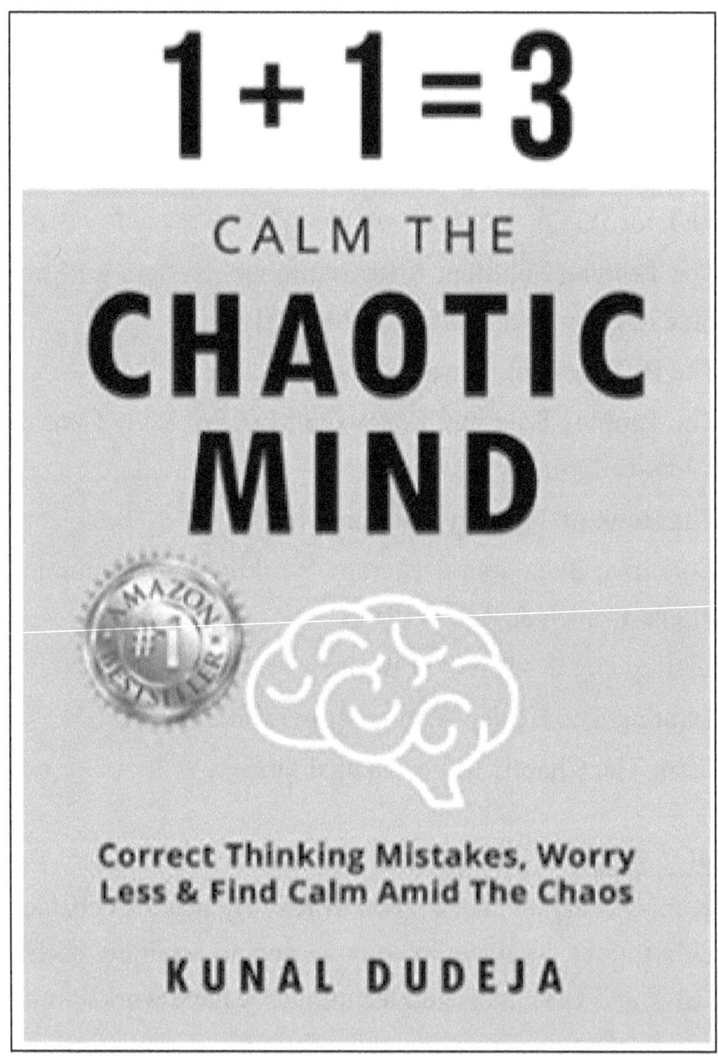